Brief Dynamic
Interpersonal Therapy

Brief Dynamic Interpersonal Therapy
A Clinician's Guide

Alessandra Lemma

Unit Director,
Psychological Therapies Development Unit,
Tavistock and Portman NHS Foundation Trust,
Visiting Professor,
Psychoanalysis Unit,
University College London, and
Visiting Professor, Essex University

Mary Target

Professor of Psychoanalysis,
University College London, and
Professional Director, Anna Freud Centre

Peter Fonagy

Freud Memorial Professor,
University College London, and
Chief Executive, Anna Freud Centre

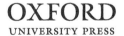

OXFORD
UNIVERSITY PRESS

OXFORD
UNIVERSITY PRESS

Great Clarendon Street, Oxford OX2 6DP
United Kingdom

Oxford University Press is a department of the University of Oxford.
It furthers the University's objective of excellence in research, scholarship,
and education by publishing worldwide. Oxford is a registered trade mark of
Oxford University Press in the UK and in certain other countries

Published in the United States of America by Oxford University Press
198 Madison Avenue, New York, NY 10016, United States of America

British Library Cataloguing in Publication Data
Data available

Library of Congress Cataloging in Publication Data
Data available

ISBN 978-0-19-960245-2

Whilst every effort has been made to ensure that the contents of this work,
are as complete, accurate and up-to-date as possible at the date of writing,
Oxford University Press is not able to give any guarantee or assurance that
such is the case. Readers are urged to take appropriately qualified medical
advise in all cases. The information in this work is intended to be useful to the
general reader, but should not be used as a means of self-diagnosis or for the
prescription of medication.

To our parents and children

Preface—Do We Need Dynamic Interpersonal Therapy?

We are short of neither psychodynamic therapies nor acronyms. Inevitably, by developing dynamic interpersonal therapy (DIT), we have added to an already long list. A reasonable question is why, then, have we done this? This question is especially pertinent because DIT's techniques and theoretical underpinnings are not novel and will be very familiar to psychodynamically trained practitioners. We are therefore not offering any new techniques or understandings, which might be regarded as a less than engaging way to start a book about DIT. But we are indeed very clear that we never set out with the intention to develop a "new" model of psychodynamic therapy as such. Rather, we present DIT as a protocol that will hopefully assist psychodynamically trained clinicians to *work to a specific focus* relevant to the difficulties commonly encountered by patients with depression and/or anxiety. More specifically, DIT strives to achieve this within a time limit (set at sixteen sessions within this protocol) that fits in with the demands placed on the provision of psychodynamic therapy within the public healthcare system, and increasingly too in the private sector where brief interventions are in high demand. DIT therefore provides a way of delineating a particular focus for intervention rather than representing a distinctively new model of therapy.

As an approach DIT is *interpersonal* because it focuses squarely on the patient's relationships, internal and external, as they relate to the problem(s) in the patient's current life, giving rise to symptoms of depression and/or anxiety. An interpersonal focus is shared with several other modalities, not least interpersonal psychotherapy (IPT) (Weissman et al., 2000), with which, somewhat confusingly, it also shares some of its title. Yet the "interpersonal" in DIT is important because it clearly sets it apart from those dynamic models that focus more on intrapsychic variables. Unlike IPT, which does not address internalized object-relationships, DIT systematically focuses on the activation in the present of one selected internalized, often unconscious, object-relationship that is meaningfully linked to the presenting problems.

DIT is *dynamic* in its focus in so far as it is concerned with helping the patient to understand the interplay between external and internal reality as it relates to a problematic circumscribed relational pattern. Consequently it addresses a nonconscious realm of experience, which again distinguishes DIT from IPT, and closely aligns it with other psychodynamic models.

Although there is substantive overlap between DIT and other psychodynamic models, for clinicians trained in long-term psychodynamic therapy or counseling implementing DIT will, most likely, feel unfamiliar as it is indeed rather different in some respects. It is "different" in so far as the therapeutic priorities singled out in DIT are not typically ones that are taught in the context of intensive psychodynamic trainings though they may well turn out to be the ones utilized by "good" therapists irrespective of the planned length of therapy (Binder, 2004).

Most psychoanalytic trainings provide the foundations for open-ended, often intensive, interventions. And yet, once qualified, many therapists find themselves working briefly without a framework to orient them to the task in hand when a time limit is imposed. Consequently the transition between long-term, intensive work to time-limited, once-weekly therapy is not always a smooth one. However experienced we are in long-term work, we cannot simply export strategies that are helpful in that context with unselected patient groups, and apply them in a brief context without any modifications. DIT has indeed been developed primarily for pragmatic reasons so that clinicians with a psychodynamic psychotherapy or counseling training can readily acquire the specific priorities and competences associated with time-limited therapeutic work with depressed and/or anxious patients.

The *application* of psychoanalytic theory and techniques to deliver a brief therapy is sometimes unhelpfully conflated with a dilution of psychoanalysis and, as such, is seen as not *really* psychoanalytic—the creation of a bastard offspring of the so-called "real thing." Such adaptations seem to arouse the doubt that psychoanalysis will be damaged by the intrusion of other ways of theorizing, thinking and practicing that may be felt to be demolishing the original edifice. Integration and adaptation may be presented as development, but experienced as undermining (Lemma and Johnston, 2010).

Preserving the "gold" of psychoanalysis was a core aim in the early days of the psychoanalytic movement (Kirsner, 1990), and this sentiment is not entirely absent from current debates about psychoanalysis and its applications in the public sector. The development of a brief intervention is sometimes construed as yet another nail in the coffin of long-term psychoanalysis, as if the existence of the briefer alternative means that this is the one that will always be selected over the longer-term, more expensive option. In the public health sector costs can, and do, drive decision making in unhelpful ways. But the eradication of long-term, intensive analytic work is not a hidden agenda that has driven the development of DIT. On the contrary, we are clear that DIT has been developed for use with a very particular patient population, in a particular public healthcare context (though this does not preclude its use in the private sector), and that patients with personality disorders, for example, would not benefit from this type of brief intervention as it stands. Having said this, sixteen sessions of DIT in a primary care context might well help some patients to identify the need for further therapy and be better able to use it than if referred directly to a less structured, open-ended psychodynamic therapy, which might prove too challenging/demanding of the patient.

To keep alive the invaluable contribution that psychoanalysis can make to public mental health, and for it to take up its legitimate place within a modern healthcare economy, it is vital that it adapts and evolves to meet the diverse needs of the patients who seek help nowadays (Lemma and Patrick, 2010). This is not about diluting the "real thing," rather, it is about development, which inevitably also brings with it change and hence loss. Not engaging in this process of adaptation and change only serves to marginalize psychoanalysis further in what has undeniably become an inhospitable external climate to psychoanalytic interventions. This protocol is but one small initiative aimed at supporting psychodynamic therapy in such a climate and sits alongside other such initiatives in the UK and elsewhere that have inspired us.

Alessandra Lemma
Mary Target
Peter Fonagy

Acknowledgments

Every idea or new development is only made possible by those that precede it. The development of DIT owes a huge debt to the work of many colleagues who developed the treatment manuals that provided the basis for the competence framework for the practice of psychodynamic psychotherapy, which underpins the development of DIT for mood disorders. We expect that our colleagues will find many areas of overlap, certainly technically, and sometimes theoretically too, with their own versions of psychodynamic therapy.

We would also like to extend our deep gratitude to the team of clinicians who were involved in our original pilot study. Their experience of implementing DIT in a primary care context has been invaluable and has contributed to the refinements we have been able to make to it. In particular we would like to thank Tamara Gellman, Jane Gibbons, Lucy Marks, Anne McKay and Pauline O'Hanlon, who all saw patients using DIT and contributed some of the clinical examples in this book, and to Mary Burd, who as then Head of the Tower Hamlets Primary Care Psychology Service generously welcomed us and supported this initiative. Finally, we are grateful to Dr Richard Taylor for sharing so generously and enthusiastically his reflections on his experience of training in DIT.

Contents

Abbreviations

BPT	brief psychodynamic therapy
CAT	cognitive analytic therapy
CBT	cognitive behavioral therapy
DBT	dialectical behavior therapy
DIT	dynamic interpersonal therapy
EBM	evidence-based medicine
fMRI	functional magnetic resonance imaging
GAD	generalized anxiety disorder
IN	interpersonal narrative
IPAF	interpersonal-affective focus
ISTDP	intensive short-term dynamic psychotherapy
IWMs	internal working models
LTPP	long-term psychodynamic psychotherapy
MBT	mentalization-based therapy
MDD	major depressive disorder
NICE	National Institute of Health and Clinical Excellence
NNT	number needed to treat
OCD	obsessive-compulsive disorder
PD	personality disorder
PTSD	post-traumatic stress disorder
RCT	randomized controlled trial
RDoC	Research Domain Criteria
SAEs	spontaneous adverse events
SCM	structured clinical management
SSRIs	selective serotonin reuptake inhibitors
STPP	short-term psychodynamic psychotherapy
TAU	treatment as usual

Chapter 1

Dynamic Interpersonal Therapy: New Wine in an Old Bottle?

In this chapter we contextualize the development of DIT in the climate of evidence-based practice, which has been broadly hostile to psychodynamic interventions. We outline the rationale for the development of this protocol in the work on developing competence frameworks and the Improving Access to Psychological Therapies initiative in the UK. Finally we review its theoretical origins in attachment theory, object relations theory and Harry Stack Sullivan's interpersonal psychoanalysis.

Evidence-based practice and the fate of psychodynamic psychotherapy

Research and psychoanalysis have not enjoyed a comfortable relationship. However, in the current climate of the public health sector they need to become better acquainted with each other because evidence-based practice, as a primary driver in healthcare, is here to stay. We have to engage with the demand this places on us as providers of psychodynamic psychotherapy and demonstrate that what we offer can make a distinctive, effective contribution to public mental health. The demand for public accountability urges us, with unprecedented force, to consider whether we want the psychoanalytic body of knowledge and its applications to be a relic of historical interest or at the cutting edge of mental healthcare.

Engagement with this demand requires that we try out different ways of doing things, which may feel alien to established practice (e.g. session-by-session outcome monitoring as is required in dynamic

interpersonal therapy [DIT]), and to many may seem altogether irrelevant to what transpires in the therapeutic situation. Arguably this
also requires that we actively respond to this external culture from a
vantage point that is distinctively psychoanalytic and practice-based
so that we are not just "complying" with what we feel is imposed on
us (though sometimes we have to do that too, of necessity). We also
need to contribute to the discourse about the varieties of scientific
research, and the contributions and limitations of different kinds of
methodologies.

In this section we will briefly review the evidence base for long-term
and brief psychodynamic interventions and what we can learn from it.
Along the way we also point out some of the limitations of the meas-
urements and methodologies used, and hence of the evidence base
itself.

The origins of psychotherapy research[1]

Over half a century ago Eysenck (1952) made the claim that psychotherapy worked no better than the facility nature gave all of us to
recover from psychological disturbance by a process of spontaneous
healing. This claim profoundly challenged the beliefs held by the
advocates of psychotherapy in general and it was responded to with a
concerted research effort, over many years, to study the effectiveness
of psychotherapy. Over time these efforts have yielded an "evidence
base" that shows, after all, that psychotherapy (in its generic sense)
does work, with the average effect size of psychotherapy found to be
0.8 across probably over 1,000 studies (Wampold, 2001). Effect size
(ES) refers to the likelihood that a person treated with psychotherapy
would be better off than a person in the control group if both were
chosen at random (Cohen, 1962).

An effect size[2] of 0.8 for psychotherapy versus no therapy is BIG—in
a moderate sort of way (Wampold et al., 2007). It means that nearly

---

[1] This section is a substantially revised version of the paper by P. Fonagy (2010).
[2] An effect size of less than 0.3 is too close to the 50 percent mark (i.e., too close to
   chance) to call it a significant effect. From 0.3 (where 58 percent of those treated
   are better off than untreated controls) to 0.6 (where two-thirds are better off) the
   effect is considered weak. From 0.6 to 0.9 (where three-quarters of those treated

three-quarters of patients who have psychotherapy are better off than those left to recover by themselves. As a marker, for those who take aspirin as a prophylaxis for heart attacks, the number needed to treat (NNT) before you see one unequivocal case that benefited is 129. For psychotherapy this figure is 3. The effect size for psychotherapy is thus superior to almost all interventions in cardiology, geriatric medicine, asthma, flu vaccines, and cataract surgery. Psychotherapy is mostly as effective as psychoactive medication and there is evidence that additional benefit accrues from combining the two in some contexts (e.g. Cuijpers et al., 2008).

The problem with effect sizes, however, is that they are inherently ambiguous: a treatment could attain a moderate effect size by producing a very LARGE EFFECT for a SMALL SUBSET of patients, or achieving a moderate but incomplete reduction in symptoms for many. To clarify this, psychotherapy researchers have collected data on the percentage recovered or percentage improved both by some predefined criterion. Drew Westen and Elizabeth Bradley (Westen and Bradley, 2005) have provided us with an impressive meta-analysis of six disorders—major depressive disorder (MDD), panic disorder, generalized anxiety disorder (GAD), obsessive-compulsive disorder (OCD), bulimia nervosa and post-traumatic stress disorder (PTSD)—based on percentage improvers. They tell a sobering tale. Whilst across disorders, treatment versus control effect sizes tend to be moderate or large, on average only roughly half of patients who *complete* treatments in these trials improve substantially. The figures are even more sobering when we compute the percentage of those who improved on the basis of all those who *entered* treatment. On average, only 33 percent of those who

---

are better than untreated controls) effect sizes are thought of as medium and beyond 0.9 we are in the land of strong effect sizes. Effect sizes are sometimes used to describe the change between the beginning and the end of a trial (pre–post effect size) and the difference between a treated and an untreated group at termination (between group effect size). Pre–post effect sizes combine the effect of treatment with the "monster" that Eysenck raised—spontaneous remission. One final note about the language of researchers is that differences are expressed in terms of the number of individuals who need to be treated before we come upon a person who unequivocally would not have got better on their own without the treatment (Laupacis et al., 1988).

entered treatment for depression can expect to improve significantly based on these figures.

Not surprisingly, improvement rates relate to severity and treatment duration (Kopta et al., 1999). On average, acute distress improves in three-quarters of cases within 25 sessions. But chronic disorders, defined in various ways, appear to require longer-term treatment. There is a less than 60 percent improvement rate after 25 sessions. The situation is even worse for those who receive what we might refer to as a complex disorder diagnosis, that is, three or more diagnoses or a diagnosis of a personality disorder (PD). Here improvement rates are less than 40 percent after 25 sessions. There is even some indication of inadvertent harm being done to patients with some PDs if they are offered time-limited treatment, so that they end up worse off than when they started (Tyrer et al., 2004).

Recent work carefully following a group of patients with private healthcare insurance, reported that about one-and-a-half years of treatment was required before the average patient achieved an acceptable level of improvement (Puschner et al., 2007). Incidentally, this work found no evidence for the much cited exponential rate of improvement originally demonstrated by Ken Howard (Howard et al., 1986). Rather, the relationship between improvement and time is best illustrated by a straight line.

The demise of the randomized controlled trial

Over the last couple of decades the randomized controlled trial (RCT) has been held by many to be the gold standard in psychotherapy research (Sackett et al., 2000; Strauss et al., 2005). Its advocates swear allegiance to evidence-based medicine (EBM) as "the conscientious explicit and judicious use of current best evidence in making decisions about the care of individual patients" (Sackett et al., 1996). Their slogans are motivational, persuasive, and essentialist rather than reportive, stipulative, and operational. The initiative is basically synonymous with attempts experimentally to establish a causal relationship between treatment and outcome.

In 2008 Sir Michael Rawlins, the Director of the National Institute of Health and Clinical Excellence (NICE), gave a Harveian Oration at the Royal College of Physicians about the overvaluation of RCTs in EBM (Rawlins, 2008). He pointed out that frequently such trials are inappropriate. There can be bioethical and legal problems in randomizing people to ineffective or harmful treatments. Some conditions are so rare and some treatment effects so great that few would consider RCTs to be sensible. For example, parachutes are very widely used despite the fact that they have not been subjected to RCTs. He also pointed out that the null hypothesis of RCTs was there often for show rather than genuine conviction. It was certainly inappropriate where previous studies had already shown an effect and statistically and conceptually difficult if the aim of the study was to show no difference between treatment arms. Rawlins also identified some challenges in relation to applying theories of probability in RCTs.

Many studies use multiple variables to measure outcome, and this can create a great deal of confusion. A study of reviews of the value of selective serotonin reuptake inhibitors (SSRIs) for pediatric depression (Fonagy and Higgitt, 2009) revealed that there are only about 15 RCTs but nearly 100 reviews have been published since 2005. These review the same investigations but come to dramatically different conclusions by focusing on different aspects of the results reported in the original investigations. The conclusions vary anywhere from "ban all SSRIs" to "use SSRIs as first line of treatment" with various gradations in between.

Sir Rawlins went on to revisit the issue most frequently alluded to in considering the appropriateness of RCTs in psychotherapy: how generalizable are the results of RCTs? Certainly, the settings in which psychotherapy RCTs take place are quite different from the real clinical situation (La Greca et al., 2009; Weiss et al., 2009). Most are undertaken in well-specified populations over a relatively brief period of time. Real-life psychotherapy is offered to heterogenous groups presenting with comorbidity that would exclude them from RCTs. Even if they might be included they often decline participation. Certainly patients in trials and "real life" differ in age, gender, severity, risk factors, comorbidities, ethnicity, and socioeconomic status. As if that was not bad enough, the treatment given in psychotherapy RCTs rarely fits clinical reality in terms of dose (frequency of therapy), timing of administration, duration of therapy, intercurrent treatments, and the skills and commitment of the practitioners. There are major differences in the setting, the way the therapists are reimbursed, and their professional priorities—publication versus clinical care. There is therefore a real question about whether the assessment of benefit obtained from a trial can be applied to ordinary clinical settings.

The assessment of harm is yet another problem: RCTs are very poor at testing for the possibility of harm (e.g., Lilienfeld, 2007; Roback, 2000). Jefferys et al. (1998) noted that surveying drugs introduced between 1972 and 1994, they could find 22 that were withdrawn for safety reasons, but only one withdrawn for lack of efficacy. This is hardly surprising, as RCTs are rarely powered up to scrutinizing adverse events. The controversy over SSRIs and pediatric suicide is a good example. None of the placebo-controlled trials are large enough to show a significant difference in rates of spontaneous adverse events (SAEs). When taken together, they showed such events to be twice as frequent amongst children and adolescents taking active medication rather than placebo. But then those advocating the use of these drugs argue that the study designs and samples are too heterogeneous to permit that kind of integration.

So perhaps, as Rawlins concluded, the advocates of RCTs have been inappropriately elevated above those conducting observational studies. The hierarchy is illusory. Both kinds of study have advantages and disadvantages. In making decisions about cost-effective treatments against a background of limited resources, we need to appraise all the evidence and *exercise judgment*. RCTs are enormously costly. They are not only resource-intensive in terms of money—they also take up considerable time and energy. Perhaps it is for this reason that their reporting is so often troubled by bias, aiming to emphasize the differences and being relatively silent about null findings. Take just one recent example on therapy for treatment-resistant depression in adolescents (Brent et al., 2008). Reading the abstract of this study we learn that when a young person did not respond to at least one SSRI, 40 percent are likely to improve if offered a medication switch. But they will improve even more if this switch is accompanied by cognitive behavioral therapy (CBT). The response rate increase is 15 percent. It makes no difference if they are switched to another SSRI or venlafaxine, but adding a psychological treatment clearly improves response rate.

A disturbingly large number of young people withdrew from each arm of the treatment (out of 334 randomized, 102—almost one third—withdrew from the treatment, a significant number [41] because of adverse events). This raises real concerns about the acceptability of any of the treatment arms. Looking at responders, it seems clear that adding CBT improved response rates, although this seems less clear when we look at only those young people who completed the treatment trial (i.e., had the full benefit of CBT).

The story here is about something else, far more serious in relation to EBM, and well-illustrated by this study. It is about three figures, which one of us (PF) drew on the basis of numbers reported in very large, hard to access tables in the journal. These concerned children's self-report of depression, suicidal ideation, and the global assessment of independent observers. It is very difficult to see any difference whatsoever between the severity of depression, suicidal ideation, or even the probably not-so-blind assessors' rating of global functioning. The conclusion reported by the researchers is that the combination of CBT and a switch to another antidepressant results in "a higher rate of clinical response than did medication switch alone." In the body of the paper, which is all about the value of CBT for this group, there is a telling sentence: "There were no differential treatment effects on scalar measures of depression, suicidal ideation, and functioning, nor were there treatment effects on suicide attempts, or self-harm-related measures" (Brent et al., 2008: 911).

Many other similar examples of biased reporting of results could be brought to bear; they are more common in the pharmacological literature, where commercial interests are great, but they are by no means unique to them. Nor would we wish to suggest that psychodynamic researchers are any less hampered by self-serving biases than those from other orientations. Years ago one of our champion researchers, Lester Luborsky published an entertaining paper that showed how we could magically divine the conclusion of a paper on psychotherapeutic outcome just by knowing the theoretical orientation of its first author (Luborsky et al., 1999). Our point here is that notwithstanding the rhetoric of EBM, conscientious, explicit, and judicious it frequently is not. As psychotherapists we understand how the mind has ways of distorting reality to maximize pleasure and minimize psychic pain.

Those energetically in pursuit of making conscientious, explicit, and judicious use of current evidence are unlikely to be any different from the rest of us. The moral has to be: "Read carefully, don't believe everything you do read and look for things that could and should be there."

Long-term psychodynamic psychotherapy (LTPP)

The RCT may be overrated but these and other research efforts have nevertheless made it possible to accumulate a good evidence base for the efficacy of psychological therapies. Over 1,000 studies demonstrate that in relation to major mental health conditions they can achieve significant symptom reductions and in some cases, particularly with anxiety disorders, freedom from symptoms. They can help to improve social adjustment and work relationships. This encouraging picture is a general one, however: there are many different types of psychological therapy and some commonly used ones have been less well researched than others. There is, as we know, more evidence for CBT than for psychodynamic psychotherapy. Of course, absence of evidence is not evidence of ineffectiveness. Moreover there is *some* evidence and we will review this now.

LTPP has posed a greater challenge to researchers, not least because of the problem of randomization, which involves getting the patients' agreement to go without the preferred treatment for 18 months or more. Finding an appropriate control group is itself a challenge, as is the blinding of assessors, and the creation of manuals to guide work over a lengthy time period and ensure that what takes place corresponds to what is described (i.e., treatment integrity). Yet for psychoanalytic clinicians this is the Holy Grail. It is long-term treatment that many of us have been trained to do and that we wish to make claims for.

It is nothing short of miraculous that enough data have been collected for two prestigious systematic reviews to have been published (Gerber et al., 2010; Leichsenring and Rabung, 2008). A review by de Maat et al. (2009) collected together 27 studies where the impact of long-term therapy on symptom reduction was measured and/or information on personality changes was collected. The unmet challenge of the control groups meant that effect sizes were pre-post, not between-group. Nevertheless, the studies covered the treatment of over 5,000 patients. The effect sizes of outcome measures combined were between 0.8 and 1 and tended, if anything, to slightly increase on follow-up and were somewhat bigger for psychoanalysis than psychotherapy. The percentage success rate on symptoms was around 70 percent based on clinicians' opinion and between 60 and 70 percent for patient self-report, when success was defined as at least moderate improvement.

The Leichsenring meta-analysis was very ambitious and identified 23 studies. The studies concerned difficult problems, but pre-post effect sizes were consistently large. For chronic problems, the effect size was 0.87–2.45, for complex depression and anxiety it was 0.97–1.94, multiple problems 0.94–1.84, and PD 0.82–1.65. Controversially, the authors contrasted these effects with those normally obtained for similar client groups in short-term therapy and found a significant superiority for long-term treatment. The size of effects varied according to type of measure, with the largest effect sizes consistently obtained on target problems, and social and personality functioning coming some way behind. However, the effects were consistently positive, with the confidence interval around the effect sizes comfortably above the line of insignificance.

As you might imagine, this news did not remain unchallenged for long (Beck and Bhar, 2009; Glass, 2008; Kriston et al., 2009; Roepke and Renneberg, 2009; Thombs et al., 2009) and the ensuing correspondence had the consistent theme of challenging positive evidence for long-term treatment. The details should perhaps be consigned to the history books, but the points raised address the nature both of the original studies (the review was based on studies with small samples with a likely bias towards the positive, treating a wide range of disorders with poorly specified control groups, and uncontrolled for contact and the structure of treatment) and of the methodology of the review (conflating within-group and between-group effect sizes, selective inclusion and exclusion of studies, etc.).

The substance of the criticisms was hard to deny. Many of the studies reviewed were in effect uncontrolled and heterogeneous and it is hard to feel confident that the original critique by Eysenck was adequately addressed by the original collection of reports. In a subsequent study that tried to respond to these criticisms, they identified

10 controlled studies of LTPP versus other types of treatment (Bachar et al., 1999; Bateman and Fonagy, 1999; Bateman and Fonagy, 2008; Clarkin et al., 2007; Dare et al., 2001; Gregory et al., 2008; Huber et al., submitted; Korner et al., 2006; Svartberg et al., 2004) where these treatments were used in the treatment of complex disorders, chiefly PD (7), eating disorders (2), and depression (1). The comparisons are with CBT, dialectical behavior therapy (DBT), cognitive analytic therapy (CAT), structured clinical management (SCM), and treatment as usual (TAU). The treatments lasted on average 70 weeks offering 120 sessions. The comparison treatments lasted about the same time, although they offered fewer sessions. The findings were similar to the previous analysis. The average between-group effect size was 0.67, somewhat larger for target problems, 0.88, than general psychiatric symptoms, 0.54. Medium effect size differentiated the comparison groups from LTPP in terms of personality and social function.

Why are these findings of enormous importance? This is the first set of strong signals that suggests that LTPP is superior to less intensive treatments when directed towards complex mental disorders. But whilst it is reassuring and helpful that LTPP therapists struggle for longer and ultimately more effectively than is the case in other modalities, we do not know how well a CBT therapist would do if they also saw their patients over long periods of time. Moreover the LTPP therapists obtained good outcomes with suicidal self-harming female patients (both borderline personality disorder (BPD) and eating disorder samples are 80 percent female). But how common are such challenges in our consulting rooms where we take the same amount of time, and sometimes longer, to rescue individuals of both genders, who perhaps, at least superficially, are in less distress? Is the superiority of LTPP still evident, and if so in what respect? The study of private insurance cases (Puschner et al., 2007) would suggest caution: when psychoanalytic psychotherapy and psychodynamic psychotherapy were tracked over 2 years in 480 patients no significant differences were seen in the rate or extent of decline between these two groups.

The most ambitious study of psychoanalytic psychotherapy comes from Helsinki (Knekt et al., 2008). It contrasted solution-focused therapy and psychodynamic psychotherapy with LTPP for patients with mixed depression and anxiety problems. The patients were followed up over 3 years. This was just as well because significant benefit from long-term treatment was not found at 18 months, nor even at 24 months but *only* at 36 months. In fact the therapists who had been trained in long-term therapy took their time to achieve success and were struggling to keep up with the progress of their short-term colleagues over the first year of the trial. But of course it could be said that the patients who selected themselves for long-term treatment were the tougher customers.

Probably the best study of LTPP carried out so far is from the Munich group of Dorothea Huber and Gunter Klug (Huber et al., submitted). It is remarkable for being the only one to use a specifically psychoanalytically oriented outcome measure, Wallerstein's Scales of Psychological Functioning (Klug and Huber, 2009). The instrument is based on psychoanalytic experts' definitions and includes 17 dimensions, each divided into 2 sub-dimensions, (a) exaggerated and (b) inhibited functioning. So impulse regulation may be pathological because of overindulgence or over-inhibition. You could finally see the benefits of psychoanalysis on this measure, but even here, convincingly only after a 1-year wait. So, it seems that in looking at intensive long-term treatment we are probably measuring the wrong things and not for long enough.

Brief psychodynamic therapy (BPT) or short-term psychodynamic psychotherapy (STPP)[3]

For obvious reasons—not least economic ones—there is a strong interest in STPPs from commissioners of mental health services and patients alike. This interest is to a large measure justified by a number of factors. First, meta-analytic reviews have yielded powerful pre-post effects for psychodynamic psychotherapies for depression based on both RCTs and correlational studies (Abbass, 2007; Cuijpers et al., 2008; Knekt et al., 2008). Second, systematic examinations of patient preference show STPP to be acceptable and clearly preferred to pharmacological alternatives (Dekker, 2008; Van Overwalle, 2009). Third, there

[3] These terms are used interchangeably.

is evidence of comparable effectiveness with medication (Salminen, 2008; 38) and of its capacity to increase the effectiveness of antidepressant treatment (de Maat et al., 2009), although it needs slightly longer to become clinically effective (Dekker, 2008).[4] A further RCT by Maina, Forner, and Bogetto (2005) compared STPP and supportive therapy in the treatment of a range of depressive disorders (dysthymic disorder, depressive disorder not otherwise specified, or adjustment disorder with depressed mood). This study also lacked statistical power but found at end of treatment both treated groups were superior to a wait list condition and at 6-month follow-up psychodynamic psychotherapy had greater benefit than brief supportive therapy.

Unsurprisingly perhaps significant controversy surrounds the claim that STPP is equivalent to other therapies (Driessen, 2010; Lynch, 2009; Tolin, 2010). Comparison trials show STPP to be less effective at end of therapy than other treatments regardless of study design (RCT vs cohort studies), use of predominantly supportive or expressive techniques, the quality of blinding, the use of antidepressants, gender, age, the number of sessions, severity, community vs clinic recruitment, and intent to treat vs completer analysis. Driessen et al. (2010) report that while psychodynamic psychotherapy may be better than control conditions, it appears less efficacious when compared to other treatments at termination. At follow-ups, however (3-month and 9-month) there were no significant differences.

It seems that differences between STPP and other therapies become smaller further away from termination (termination is classically recognized to cause the reemergence of the presenting problems), and there is indication of publication bias which when adjusted for (Dwal and Tweedie, 2000) removes the statistical significance of the difference between CBT and STPP. The difference may also be exaggerated by the reactivity of some measures used. In carefully reviewing quantitative

---

[4] However, with sample sizes of 25 per arm, there was insufficient statistical power to be confident of detecting differences between treatments. It should be noted that a conclusion of noninferiority requires about 90 patients per arm for even a medium size of difference ($d = 0.5$) with conventional expectations about significance levels (5 percent two-tailed) and the likelihood of missing a possible significant result (90 percent).

studies, in the light of our own qualitative reviews (Fonagy, 2005, 2010) suggesting similar conclusions, our view is that on balance the evidence favoring other therapies such as CBT and IPT over psychodynamic ones is accurate, and largely attributable to the lack of standardization and coherence in the administration of STPPs and *not* due to inherent problems with its effectiveness. For example, inferior effects from psychodynamic psychotherapy compared to CBT are observed when dynamic therapists apply methods from long-term intensive therapy in the context of short-term symptom-oriented treatments (e.g. Durham, 1994). LTPP yields substantially inferior results compared to STPP at 6 months and 1 year and shows significant advantage only after 3 years (Knekt et al., 2008). STPP is fragmented into minor submodalities focusing on "unique" features of approaches of relatively high complexity (e.g., Abbass, 2008; Kernberg et al., 2006; Malan, 2009; Neborsky, 2006) that may create artificial barriers to the acquisition of the required competencies without credible evidence to date that those features are necessary to eventual outcome for all patients (Driessen, 2010).

Relative to depression, there are not many RCTs of STPP for anxiety disorders. Milrod and colleagues (2007) have reported one small RCT of STPP for panic disorder (with or without agoraphobia) that compared psychodynamic psychotherapy with applied relaxation using a specially carefully designed manual (Milrod et al., 1997). The former was superior to the latter and the difference was particularly marked with more complex cases that had already had other failed treatments. A larger trial is currently under way. A short-term psychodynamic group therapy for generalized social phobia was found to add to the effectiveness of clonazepam and to be superior to placebo (Knijnik et al., 2008). Once again, an underpowered study (Bögels et al., 2003) reported in conference proceedings found no difference in the effectiveness of STPP and CBT in the treatment of generalized social phobia. There is, however, a large-scale multi-center RCT about to be reported which compares psychodynamic psychotherapy and CBT for social phobia (Leichsenring et al., 2009).

The picture in relation to GAD is less favorable to psychodynamic psychotherapy. In a small study Crits-Christoph and colleagues (2005) found STPP and supportive therapy to be equally effective on measures of anxiety, but STPP appeared more effective in terms of remission rates (Crits-Christoph et al., 2005). A far better designed study found CBT to be superior to STPP in the treatment of GAD both at the end of therapy and at the 6-month follow-up, although the difference was not evident on some of the key measures (Leichsenring et al., 2009). However, the differences may be entirely attributable to a modification of worrying in CBT but not STPP. Questionnaire items related to worrying in the self-report instruments used in the study showed the strongest differences (Leichsenring et al., 2010). An implication of this finding for STPP may be that the dynamic underpinnings of the kind of chronic self-focused concern that characterizes worrying should be addressed when encountered, that is, identified as a problem and its unconscious determinants made a focus of exploration and interpretation.

What can we conclude from this brief and rather superficial review of the literature? In general, STPP seems to be offered in a very general way to patients and there is little effort to shape a treatment to address the symptom profile of the individual seeking help. Underpinning this is the perhaps outdated assumption that symptoms are not relevant as they are surface manifestations of an unconscious conflict presumed to be underpinning them in much the same way that the manifest content of a dream may be set aside while trying to explore the latent content of the dream. Yet the analogy is evidently false and can lead to an overly generic approach to therapy where no principle is applied beyond the wish to freely explore mental contents.

Underlying the phenomenology of psychiatric disorder are unique disease mechanisms (Insel and Wang, 2010; Insel et al., 2010). These need to be explored even in the context of dynamic therapy. Thought needs to be given to how pathogenic mental processes impact on conscious and unconscious mental content. In our view the efficacy of psychodynamic psychotherapy will increase if therapeutic techniques aim to address the specific mechanisms that sustain the psychopathology of the respective disorder. An example is the work of Bateman and Fonagy (1999) on the mentalization-based treatment of BPD where the exploration of mental contents is undertaken with a view to restoring inhibited or decoupled capacity to think about mental states.

A new intellectual framework for psychoanalytic psychotherapy research

If we take stock of what we have reviewed so far we would be justified in thinking that the picture is more encouraging than at first reading. In one sense this is true because there is some evidence to support psychodynamic therapy, but not nearly enough to secure the future of psychodynamic interventions as an integral part of mental health services. This brings us to the present and the need to look back towards the future—the title of a brilliant paper by Patrick Luyten and Sidney Blatt (Luyten and Blatt, 2007).

If we look back at the history of psychotherapy research it becomes apparent that STPP has been competing in trials where not only the rules of engagement but also the criteria for "winning" have been defined by measuring changes that are typically responsive to medication. The outcome measures in the field of psychotherapy are self-report measures designed to be reactive to kinds of changes that neurochemical interventions promote, by and large the blunting of awareness of distress caused by symptoms. This is problematic on two counts. First, in many instances, psychodynamic psychotherapy tries to increase awareness of distress rather than reduce it. Second, it is a devastating indictment of the entire system that there has been almost no patient participation in defining outcome measures, and the entire scheme is an edifice to evidence-based practice as prescribed by professionals (Dolan et al., 2009). From a professional's standpoint, as from that of the ordinary member of the public, physical role limitation, physical function, and pain have high priority, whilst those suffering disorders rate dignity and general well-being (mood, global assessment of life, having a partner, job, lots of social contact) as more important. Well-being should feature at least alongside, if not in place of, lists of symptoms in outcome studies (Pressman and Cohen, 2005).

Measures for the most part are arbitrary, measuring subtle psychological processes on arbitrary scales, and yet we reify them, we treat them and think of them as if they correspond to something of self-evident value in the outside world (Kazdin, 2006). But what is the real life significance of change of 0.5 on the GSI score of the SCL-90?

Arbitrary or not, our measures should be neutral in relation to the nature of treatment they intend to evaluate, otherwise we might find treatments targeting the scales of measurement rather than the disease process, which of course would be a travesty.

For a number of years we have had nonreactive functional brain imaging measures of outcome available. Since Eisenberger and colleagues (2003) demonstrated that social exclusion could activate the very same brain areas (anterior cingulated cortex, right ventral prefrontal cortex) as the experience of physical pain, there have been literally hundreds of demonstrations of functional magnetic resonance imaging (fMRI) yielding accurate sensitive information related to subjective states. There have been 27 neuroimaging studies of psychotherapy using a number of imaging modalities and a range of diagnoses and therapeutic approaches (Carrig et al., 2009).

These studies have their limitations, and almost no studies provide data on changes whilst treatment is going on. However, with a little ingenuity, functional tasks could be designed which are specific not only to the disease condition, but also to the hypothesized mechanism of action of the mode of therapy. Exploring the interplay of biological and psychological processes has the potential to enhance our understanding of the mode of action of psychotherapy.

Multiple lines of evidence are likely to be needed to identify the mechanisms critical to particular types of intervention (Kazdin, 2009). The aim of this would not be to make psychological accounts redundant by providing a biological explanation, but rather to be more specific about what makes therapy work and to identify instances when it works well and for the long term.

The effectiveness research of the past 50 years, particularly the RCTs, have shown us that psychotherapy is causal in bringing about change. However, demonstrating causation is but an illusion of explanation and a pernicious illusion at that. It gives rise to superstitious behavior like Skinner's pigeons randomly delivered a pellet and thereby reinforcing whatever activity they happened to be engaged in: instead of understanding how our treatments work, we somewhat mindlessly repeat exactly the behaviors that led to the positive observed outcomes.

However, not only experimental studies but also observational studies are misleading in terms of identifying the effective components of treatments. For example, it is often claimed that the therapeutic alliance is a mediator and mechanism of therapeutic change since the stronger the alliance, the greater the change observed (Klein et al., 2003). Correlational studies also show that alliance at the beginning of treatment predicts improvement in symptoms at the end (Cloitre et al., 2004).

More recent research that contrasted the outcome of patients with a number of therapists found that differences between the effectiveness of therapists could be predicted by the strength of alliance they were likely to form with their patients (Baldwin et al., 2007), but differences in outcome between patients with the same therapist were unrelated to therapeutic alliance. If the therapeutic alliance was the mechanism of change, then we would expect to do better with patients with whom we form a good alliance than those with whom our alliance is relatively poor. This turns out spectacularly not to be the case. So the ability to form an alliance does mark out our more talented therapists, but what it is that they do more or less of that makes them more or less effective still remains a mystery.

Understanding why therapy works will increasingly require an understanding of the moderators of therapeutic effectiveness. Rapidly advancing biological research is providing persuasive evidence that there may be genetic limitations on how well therapy can work. Freud (1937), in his last major paper "Analysis Terminable and Interminable," seemed to be acutely aware of the limitations of his technique, although he might understandably have misperceived some of the processes involved. Six years ago, in a widely quoted study, Avshalom Caspi and Terri Moffitt showed that the association between the number of stressful life events an individual experienced between 21 and 26 years and the probability of depression, suicidal ideation, and suicide attempts was moderated by the 5HTT genotype (Caspi et al., 2003). Only those who had two of the short alleles of this genotype were likely to respond to four life events with increased suicidal ideation. The association between life events and suicidal ideation of those with two long alleles was completely absent.

This area of research has become a minor cottage industry, although many geneticists are appropriately skeptical about it (Risch et al., 2009). The most challenging finding for those of us aligned to attachment theory is the report from Kochanska's laboratory demonstrating that maternal sensitivity predicted infant security of attachment as it is supposed to *only* in infants with the short allele of the 5HTT genotype (Barry et al., 2008). Infants with the long allele were equally likely to be secure regardless of maternal sensitivity. Along similar lines but with older children, Kaufman reported that the depressogenic effects of maltreatment could be mitigated by social support in individuals with the short allele of the *5HTT* gene (Kaufman et al., 2004).

We are not suggesting that psychotherapy should only be offered to people without this or that allele, but rather that the mechanism by which therapy achieves its effect may be quite different for these constitutionally distinguishable groups of individuals. If we choose to ignore the reality of these differences in our clinical work, future generations are likely to judge this decision as unethical and unjustifiable and potentially as an indication of self-serving attitudes.

Conclusions

All knowledge is subject to both rational and irrational forces. It is vital to counter some of the more simplistic notions about the status of scientific findings. Equally, however, if all knowledge is vulnerable to unconscious forces this alerts us to the fact that our "clinical knowledge" is similarly compromised so that from whatever perspective we approach the task of "understanding" a phenomenon we invariably need another perspective to act as a kind of corrective. Research can provide one such "other" perspective for the clinician, just as the clinician can alert the researcher to potential blind spots in his or her scientific field of vision.

Research is there not simply to defend the boundaries of our existing domains, but to help us deliver the most efftective forms of care for our patients. To do this we have to understand better what causal mechanisms play a role in achieving patient benefit and also what circumstances can interfere with a treatment's effectiveness. Science, particularly neuroscience, will give us better ideas about how we can help our patients in more differentiated ways as it evolves.

But practice is also essential for science. Practice has to tell researchers where knowledge is most needed and to ensure that science is firmly grounded in everyday clinical care. Best evidence is only meaningful if used in proper argumentation. Argumentation is only meaningful if based on the best evidence in its building blocks. Jules Henri Poincaré wrote: "Science is built up with facts as a house is with stone, but a collection of facts is no more a science than a heap of stones is a house."

The rationale for developing DIT

The culture of EBM, as we have seen, has subjected the providers of psychodynamic psychotherapy to the requirement to justify the effectiveness of this mode of therapy. For various reasons these demands, historically, have been difficult to meet, not least because of the unfamiliarity with this more instrumental way of thinking to many psychodynamic clinicians who typically are also not trained to appraise or undertake research (Rustin, 2010).

This culture may understandably be felt to be the "enemy," as it were, of psychodynamic practice, but as well as posing a threat it has, in fact, also helpfully focused our attention not only on the importance of systematically evaluating what we do so as to monitor the quality of what we offer to patients, but also on the thorny question of therapists' competence: how we define it, hone it, and assess it.

In the UK, for example, the Department of Health has invested in the development of competences for a range of psychological therapies, including psychodynamic psychotherapy, as the basis for the development of National Occupational Standards (NOS) for the practice of psychological therapies. The origins of DIT lie in this work.

Our rationale for developing DIT is based on our collective experience as clinicians, trainers, and researchers, which persuaded us that the competence framework provided an opportunity to develop a protocol that integrates core, shared psychodynamic principles and techniques grounded in the extant evidence base, and that thus carries some external or empirical credibility when applied with a specific focus on mood disorders (depression and anxiety). DIT thus deliberately uses methods taken from across the board of dynamic therapies and we would therefore expect those who have been involved in the development of other brief dynamic models to find many familiar strategies and techniques in DIT.

In the context of modern healthcare, uncritically inherited parameters of psychodynamic practice can yield disappointing results. There is urgent need for coherent psychodynamic practice protocols that promote the rapid translation of psychological insight into symptom change, while taking full advantage of scientific progress in understanding generic principles of behavior change and incorporating these into a generic and pragmatic therapy.

DIT was designed to optimize the practical fit between a psychodynamic approach and the symptom focus of modern commissioners and consumers of psychological therapy services without compromising its theoretical tradition and its unique mechanisms of therapeutic action (Abbass, 2008; Kernberg et al., 2006; Malan, 2009; Neborsky, 2006). It was constructed to make optimal use of the basic skills of individuals with a generic psychodynamic background (Norcross, 2002; Secretary of State for Health, 2008) by offering a brief additional training in a standardized evidence-guided intervention that optimizes compatibility with current NHS practice and permits the ready evaluation of competence, adherence, and integrity.

DIT is thus not intended to be a further new psychodynamic submodality. Rather, it is a treatment and training manual compiling key elements from implementations of psychodynamic psychotherapy recognized by NICE as contributing to its evidence base (e.g. de Maat, et al. 2009; Dekker, 2008; Salminen, 2008).[5]

The Psychodynamic Competences Framework (Lemma et al., 2008)[6,7] describes a model of psychodynamic competences based on empirical evidence of efficacy. It indicates the various areas of

---

[5] In fact, 23 psychodynamic treatment trials for depression have been conducted (Driessen, 2010) although various, mostly nonoverlapping, limitations have rightly prevented their consideration by NICE guideline development groups.

[6] The full list of competences can be accessed at www.ucl.ac.uk/CORE.

[7] The Improving Access to Psychological Therapies (IAPT) programme in the UK, which was launched in May 2007, provided the backdrop for the first wave of work on the development of competences for the practice of psychological therapies. The CBT competence model was specifically developed to be a "prototype" for articulating the competences associated with other psychological therapies (Roth and Pilling, 2008).

activity that, taken together, represent what has been proven to be good clinical practice as observed in outcome trials.

This work began by identifying those psychodynamic approaches with the strongest claims for evidence of efficacy, based on the outcome in controlled trials where a manual was available. In order to determine which studies to select, the reviews of psychological therapies conducted by Roth and Fonagy (2005) were combined with the trial and systematic review database held at the Center for Outcomes, Research and Effectiveness, as part of scoping work for NICE. From the combined lists (in conjunction with an Expert Reference Group comprising senior clinicians and researchers representative of different analytic traditions) clinical trials of appropriate quality for inclusion in the framework were identified and the manuals used in these studies were located. Only trials where a manual could be accessed were included. These manuals were then studied carefully with a focus on what the therapists were expected to do. This qualitative analysis provided the basis for the articulation of the core, specific, and meta-competences required to practice psychoanalytic psychotherapy (see Figure 1.1). These competences, where possible, were peer-reviewed by the originators of the manuals and also by an Expert Reference Group. To supplement these manuals several widely cited texts that explicate psychoanalytic terminology, and provide clear descriptions of how these concepts translate into clinical practice, were also consulted (e.g., Bateman et al., 2000; Etchegoyen, 1999; Greenson, 1967; Lemma, 2003).

Are manuals helpful?

In research trials therapist performance is typically evaluated through audio or video recordings, which are then rated. This allows researchers to monitor whether the therapists in these trials adhered to the manual. In turn, this makes it possible to be reasonably confident that if procedures are followed as set out in the manual, which has been associated with substantial clinical improvements in research trials, there should be good outcomes for future patients also.

Manuals are not used in trials because they are necessarily thought to lead to better outcomes for patients—the evidence for this is, in fact, mixed (Fonagy, 1999). But in the context of an outcome study a manual

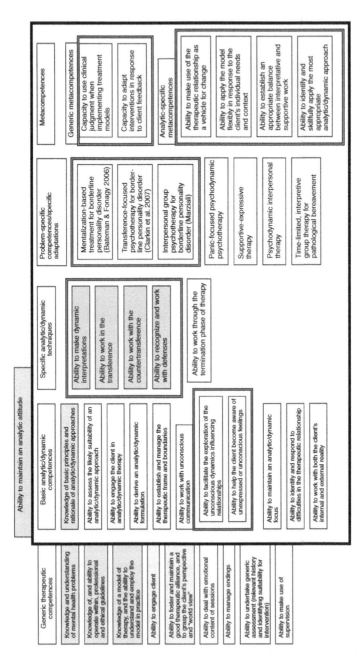

Figure 1.1 Psychodynamic/analytic competence map.

makes it possible to standardize the independent variable through reducing therapist differences (Crits-Christoph et al., 1991).

The idea of a manualized therapy often provokes varying degrees of allergic reaction from within the psychoanalytic community, raising understandable concerns about the mechanisation of the therapeutic process (e.g. Bravesmith, 2010). It is easy to see why: any attempt to somehow operationalize the therapeutic process appears at odds with the essence of the analytic attitude, which is one of the distinguishing features of an analytic approach, and its very particular kind of attunement to the complexities of the therapeutic relationship and to the inherent uncertainties encountered when attempting to understand the mind of another person.

In our view the problem is not inherent to manuals per se. Rather it depends on how they are used. The vast majority of so-called manuals—including this one—are no more than "guides" to treatment whose aim is to describe the principles of therapy in general terms consistent with the model advocated. A fundamental competence when practicing DIT is indeed the ability to implement the approach flexibly bearing in mind who the patient is (i.e., the filtering impact of personality structure on the experience of symptoms of depression or anxiety), and where in his mind, and in his external world, the patient finds himself at any given point in time during the course of a therapy. Understanding these highly idiosyncratic variables will determine how best to intervene and this may well entail going "off-manual." In this respect having the manual in mind supports a certain discipline in clinical decision making because it forces us to think explicitly about why we may decide to do something other than what is advocated in the manual.

Although in the coming chapters we present DIT as unfolding over three broad phases—an engagement and assessment phase, a middle phase, and an ending phase—and we make some suggestions about the kinds of interventions that may be helpful in each of these, we regard the therapist's *flexibility* in delivering this therapy to be the sine qua non of good clinical practice. Knowledge of therapeutic strategies and techniques does not guarantee that a therapist will be competent.

Specifying the competences required to deliver effective psychodynamic therapy

Like manuals, an exercise aimed at specifying the "competences" underpinning effective clinical practice is one known to also elicit allergic reactions since it can be seen to be reductive and irrelevant to practice. Moreover the notion of competences is unhelpfully associated with the idea of being "monitored" and the possibility that we might then be found to be incompetent.

Competence lists, like manuals, can be used rigidly and for no helpful purpose, but this does not need to be so. Indeed we have explicitly drawn on this work to provide the backbone of this protocol so as to support clinicians in monitoring what they are doing when they are practicing DIT and for what reason(s). Before outlining the specifics of DIT it is therefore important to outline the range of competences that underpin DIT as they are articulated in the competence framework.

The competence framework

The overall framework (Roth and Pilling, 2008) maps out the competences across different domains, namely generic competences, basic psychodynamic competences, specific psychodynamic techniques, and metacompetences. We will now review each of these. For ease of reference, for each of the competences we highlight the chapter(s) in this book in which each competence is addressed and discussed (see Table 1.1).

Generic competences

Although our emphasis is on working psychodynamically, the competence frameworks helpfully focus our attention on a range of generic competences that are employed in any psychological therapy, reflecting the fact that all psychological therapies, including psychodynamic therapy, share some common features. For example, therapists using any accepted theoretical model would be expected to demonstrate an ability to build a trusting relationship with their patients, relating to them in an encouraging and accepting manner. Without building a good therapist–patient relationship, technical interventions are unlikely to succeed. Often referred to as "common factors" in therapy, these competences provide an essential backdrop to the practice of psychotherapy.

Basic psychodynamic therapy competences

Basic competences establish the structure for psychodynamic therapy interventions, and form the context and structure for the implementation of a range of more specific psychodynamic techniques. For example, psychodynamic therapy prioritizes understanding the patient's unconscious experience. It is in this context that the vicissitudes of the

Table 1.1 List of psychodynamic competences

Basic psychodynamic competences
Knowledge of basic principles and rationale of dynamic approaches   Chapter 1
Ability to assess the likely suitability of a dynamic approach   Chapter 2
Ability to derive a dynamic formulation   Chapters 4, 5
Ability to establish and manage the therapeutic frame and boundaries   Chapter 4
Ability to maintain a dynamic focus   Chapters 3, 4, 5, 6
Ability to identify and respond to difficulties in the therapeutic relationship   Chapters 8, 10
Ability to work with both the client's internal and external reality   Chapter 4
Specific psychodynamic techniques
Ability to make dynamic interpretations   Chapters 5, 6, 7
Ability to work in the transference   Chapters 3, 8, 10
Ability to work with the countertransference   Chapters 8, 10
Ability to recognize and work with defenses   Chapters 5, 6,
Ability to work through the termination phase of therapy   Chapter 9
Metacompetences
Ability to make use of the therapeutic relationship as a vehicle for change   Chapters 3, 4, 5, 8, 10
Ability to apply the model flexibly in response to the client's individual needs and context   Chapters 4, 5, 7
Ability to establish an appropriate balance between interpretive and supportive work   Chapters 3, 4, 7

therapeutic relationship (i.e., the transference) are then explored. While other therapeutic modalities also attend to the therapeutic relationship, what distinguishes the psychodynamic approach is this primary focus on the patient's unconscious experience of the relationship.

Distinguishing "basic psychodynamic therapy competences" from "specific psychodynamic therapy techniques"[8]

The distinction between these domains is a very subtle one—as much pragmatic as conceptual. Essentially, "basic competences" are those deemed necessary in any dynamically informed intervention. They provide the backdrop to the more commonly applied techniques—such as working in the transference—that come under the domain of "specific techniques." Another way of thinking about the distinction is to see the basic competences as underpinning any dynamically informed therapy, whereas the use made of the specific techniques is likely to vary greatly between different psychodynamic models and their application to particular problems.

Specific psychodynamic techniques

These are the core technical interventions employed in most applications—the set of commonly applied techniques found to a lesser or greater extent in most forms of psychodynamic therapy. Examples would be the interpretation of transference and using the countertransference.

Metacompetences

A common observation is that carrying out a skilled task requires the person to be aware of why and when to do something (and just as important, when not to do it!). This is a critical skill that needs to be recognized in any competence model. Reducing psychological therapy to a series of rote operations would make little sense, because competent practitioners need to be able to implement higher-order links between theory and practice in order to plan and where necessary to adapt therapy to the needs of individual patients. These are referred

---

[8] This section is based on the original document by Lemma et al. (2008).

to as metacompetences in this framework: the procedures used by therapists to guide practice and operate across all levels of the model. These competences are more abstract than those in other domains because they usually reflect the intentions of the therapist. These can be difficult to observe directly but can be inferred from their actions, and may form an important part of discussions in supervision.

The lists are divided into two areas. Generic metacompetences are common to all therapies, and broadly reflect the ability to implement an intervention in a manner that is flexible and responsive. Psychodynamic therapy-specific metacompetences apply to the implementation of therapy in a manner that is consonant with its philosophy, as well as the way in which specific techniques are applied.

Basic psychodynamic therapy competences

This domain contains a range of activities that are basic in the sense of being fundamental areas of skill; they represent practices that underpin any psychodynamic therapy intervention.

Ability to maintain an analytic attitude Activities in all domains of psychodynamic therapy competence need to be carried out in the context of an overarching competence: the ability to approach all aspects of the interaction with the patient, and of the management of the therapeutic setting, with an "analytic attitude."

The analytic attitude describes the therapist's "position" or state of mind in relation to the work of therapy. This stance is characterized by receptiveness to the patient's unconscious communications and to the unfolding of the transference. The analytic relationship is unique in offering permissiveness of discourse: the analyst listens, but does not impose restraint, judgment, or punishment. The therapist's state of mind thus functions as "the keeper of the analytic process" (Calef and Weinschel, 1980) and so protects this privileged space.

Knowledge of the basic principles of psychodynamic therapy All psychodynamic models are more or less implicitly rooted in an assumed core knowledge base without which it would not be possible to practice psychodynamically, irrespective of the primary theoretical tradition with which we are aligned. This shared knowledge falls into three areas: knowledge of the core principles of psychodynamic therapy, of developmental theory, and of a psychodynamic model of the mind.

The ability to assess the likely suitability of psychodynamic therapy This represents a potential challenge, since we know that pre-therapy patient characteristics are not significantly predictive of outcome. Often therapists base their treatment decisions on information gleaned from the "live" experience of the assessment process and on cumulative practice-based evidence of the indications and contraindications for the approach. Psychodynamic therapy can be applied to a range of clinical problems, and a key task for any assessment is to identify those ways in which the therapy may need to be applied or adapted to meet the needs of the individual patient, as well as taking into account the resources available to the therapist (e.g. access to multidisciplinary support).

The ability to engage the patient in the therapeutic work is fundamental to any approach In psychodynamic therapy this is achieved by listening attentively and by responding nonjudgmentally to the patient's conscious and unconscious experience. It also requires that early on the therapist provides the patient with an experience of how the therapy works, for example, through maintaining the analytic attitude.

In order to engage, the patient needs to have enough information to make an informed decision about their treatment and to feel that the therapist is willing to discuss this openly with them. It is therefore important that the therapist provides the patient with direct information about the approach, including its potential risks.

The patient will also require a sense of what the therapy can help them with. An important task at this early stage involves working together with the patient to identify and agree therapeutic aims. This is particularly important when working within a time-limited frame, because a focus that is felt to be meaningful to the patient is more likely to promote engagement.

The ability to formulate This is fundamental to the practice of psychodynamic therapy even though it is often a neglected area in many trainings. The ability to formulate, and moreover to be able to do so within a few sessions, as in DIT, is essential. A formulation accounts for the developmental origins of the patient's difficulties, the underlying unconscious conflicts, the defenses associated with their management, and the recurring interpersonal patterns and expectations of others. Patients will have areas where they show a good capacity for functioning as well as areas in which they are vulnerable or have difficulties (i.e., areas of deficit and of conflict), and formulations need to reflect this balance.

Establishing and managing the therapeutic frame and boundaries This involves a range of activities and interventions, all of which are likely to have meaning for the patient. For example, changes to the time of appointments or of the therapy room can be experienced as emotionally charged events for some patients. This is why when changes or deviations occur—and they invariably do—the psychodynamic therapist works with the patient to understand the unconscious meaning the deviation has for them and helps the patient to link this with the interpersonal dynamics that are being explored in the therapy. Exploration of the patient's experience of the frame and of the boundaries of the therapeutic relationship is therefore of value in helping them to understand themselves and their difficulties.

The ability to work with unconscious communication underpins the next two areas of competence, namely facilitating the exploration of unconscious feelings and of the unconscious dynamics influencing relationships This refers to a particular quality of listening in which the explicit content of the patient's communications is considered to be the "tip of an iceberg" of reference and implication. Therapists need to take what the patient is telling them at face value, but also to be attuned to meanings which are inherent or implied. In this sense they are listening to several levels of discourse simultaneously, making this a distinctive and sophisticated skill. Of course, communication would fail if the therapist did not attend to the first level of implication of what the patient said to them; an overemphasis on what the patient is not explicitly saying can undermine the development of a good therapeutic alliance.

The primary means of unconscious communication are the patient's narratives, dreams, and their free associations (the spontaneous links they make between ideas). The therapist can facilitate unconscious communication by knowing when to allow silence, so that free associations can emerge.

The therapist listens out for recurring affective and interpersonal themes. Listening in this way is not a passive process. It involves actively being with the patient, moment-by-moment, and tracking the often subtle changes in their state of mind; this reflects the central importance of the therapist's receptivity to the patient's unconscious communications. It also points to the fact that it is impossible to listen without also being in some way personally involved. The ability to be self-reflective and to identify the need for consultation and supervision (or further personal therapy, where required) are therefore key competences.

The ability to maintain an analytic focus This refers to two distinct, but related, activities. First, it underlines that psychodynamic therapy's primary, overarching focus is on the exploration of the patient's unconscious experience. Essentially this means that all aspects of the work are approached with an analytic attitude. Second, it refers to working on a particular dynamic theme or conflict to the relative exclusion of others for the duration of the therapy. This is usually the case in time-limited therapy, as it is in DIT, where it is essential to negotiate with the patient a circumscribed conflict or interpersonal pattern that will provide direction and a boundary for both patient and therapist.

The ability to identify and manage difficulties in the therapeutic relationship Because psychodynamic approaches use the therapeutic relationship as the main vehicle for change, the ability to identify and manage difficulties within this relationship is an important skill. For example, whether an interpretation is experienced as helpful will be determined, in large part, by the patient's dominant experience of the relationship at that particular moment in time.

The ability to work with both the patient's internal and external reality Psychodynamic approaches prioritize the exploration of the patient's subjective, unconscious experience, and therapists need the ability to work with both the patient's internal and external reality. The internal world is, however, always in a dynamic interaction with the external world. To get as close as possible to the patient's experience it is therefore essential to also take into account the external reality of the patient's life. Moreover, the therapeutic relationship will also be affected by the perceived differences (e.g. of age, culture) and similarities between the patient and therapist. These need to be openly and sensitively explored, not only because these perceptions are often rich in meaning, but also because, left unexplored, they can become the source of misunderstandings between patient and therapist and can undermine the therapeutic alliance.

Specific psychodynamic therapy techniques

This domain includes the main techniques employed by psychodynamic therapists—making dynamic interpretations (particularly of the transference), making use of the countertransference, and working with defenses. Not all of these would be employed for any one individual, and different technical emphases would be deployed for different problems.

Ability to make dynamic interpretations

An interpretation puts into words the patient's conscious and unconscious experience. Often interpretations serve the function of validating the patient's experience; they convey to the patient that the therapist has understood their predicament by going one step beyond an acknowledgement of what the patient consciously feels. Sometimes an interpretation brings together disparate elements in a way that can be challenging, because it introduces a new perspective on the patient's experience. It is important therefore to create the conditions of safety within which the patient can tolerate these challenges, which are a necessary part of the therapeutic enterprise.

Ability to work with transference and countertransference

Psychodynamic therapy is a relational therapy that focuses on helping the patient to understand the dynamic factors (e.g. unconscious feelings and fantasies) that shape their behavior. It is through addressing these factors, and not simply the experiences that have contributed to them, that therapeutic change is thought to occur.

A transference interpretation makes explicit reference to the patient–therapist relationship and is intended to elucidate and encourage an exploration of the patient's conflicts as they are manifest in the relationship. Although the emphasis is not on the patient's past, work in the transference can cast light on this.

The main focus for interpretation is the patient's recurring interpersonal and affective patterns as they manifest themselves in the transference relationship. These interpretations are often referred to as "here and now" or transference. Although they can refer to figures from the patient's past, the primary focus in on the relationship with the therapist as it unfolds in the consulting room. This means that the therapist's focus is usually on the formulation and interpretation of the patient's current experience of themselves in relationship with other people.

The therapist's ability to consider the meaning and relevance of their countertransference

The ability to make use of the therapist's emotional reactions to the patient is important. This will involve monitoring their own contribution to the interaction because the quality of the relationship that evolves between the therapist and the patient is determined by unconscious forces operating in both. This therefore requires a well-honed capacity to self-monitor and to identify the therapist's own contribution to enactments.

Ability to work with defenses

All psychodynamic approaches aim to identify the nature of the patient's anxiety and how they manage this. This will involve the therapist establishing whether the defenses are directed internally (to ward off awareness of threatening thoughts and feelings) or externally (for example, avoiding intimacy with others). Often they may serve both functions.

A key task for the therapist is to identify how defenses manifest themselves in the patient's communications and ways of relating to the therapist and other people. Because defenses exist for a good reason the therapist approaches them sensitively, with due respect for the patient's need for the defenses, mindful, too, of the possibility of colluding with them.

In the therapeutic situation defenses often manifest themselves as resistances, that is, as a kind of "opposition" to the therapy. Working with resistance therefore involves helping the patient to think about the different, and often conflicting, motivations that lie beneath their wish to seek help.

Ability to work through the termination phase of therapy

Finishing therapy in a planned manner is important not only because patients (and often therapists) may have strong feelings about ending, but also because this allows for discussion of how the patient will manage on their own and what further help, if any, they might need. This process is aided by ensuring that the likely schedule for sessions is signaled from the outset, and that there is explicit discussion towards the end of therapy about the conscious and unconscious meaning of the ending for the patient.

DIT's theoretical framework

Although the techniques and strategies used in DIT reflect the findings of the competence framework for psychodynamic psychotherapy, an approach that failed to contextualize theoretically what the therapist is aiming to do and why would be very limited. Consequently we have embedded DIT in a range of psychoanalytic ideas that we consider to be highly relevant to understanding mood disorders and their impact on an individual's internal and external worlds. We hope that this framework yields enough common ground to make the model of interest to psychodynamic clinicians with a range of theoretical affiliations.

DIT's overarching principles are rooted in core psychoanalytic ideas that emphasize a number of assumptions. These assumptions not only have face validity in the clinical situation, but several of them are also supported by empirical observations (Fonagy and Target, 2003) namely:

- The impact of early childhood experiences on adult functioning, with particular attention to adult attachment processes and the significance of mental models of relationships.
- The internal and external forces that shape the mind and therefore inform our perception of ourselves in relationships with others.
- The existence of an unconscious realm of experience that is a motivating force.
- The unconscious projective and introjective processes that underpin the subjective experience of relationships.
- The ubiquity of the transference, by which patients respond to others, and to the therapist, according to developmental models that have not been updated or challenged.

Although we draw on this shared pool of overarching psychody-namic ideas we also draw more specifically on object relations theory, attachment theory, and Sullivan's interpersonal psychoanalysis.

Object-relations theory

Object-relations theory is too diverse to have an agreed definition (Kramer and Akhtar, 1988), and as object-relations theories have come to dominate psychoanalysis, most theorists have appeared to aspire to this category. Greenberg and Mitchell, in their classic over-view, use the term to include all theories "concerned with exploring the relationship between real, external people and the internal images and residues of relations with them and the significance of these resi-dues for psychic functioning" (1983: 14).

Kernberg (1976) distinguishes three uses of the term object-relations theory:

1. The understanding of present relationships in terms of past ones, which would include the study of intrapsychic structures as deriving from fixation, modifying, and reactivating earlier internalizations.

2. A specialized approach within psychoanalytic metapsychology, involving mental representations of dyadic "self"–"object" relationships, which are rooted in the original relation of the baby and mother, and the later development of this relation into dyadic, triadic, and multiple internal and external relationships.

3. Specific approaches of (a) the Kleinian school, (b) the British Independent tradition, and (c) those theorists who have attempted to integrate the ideas of these schools into their own developmental theory.

In this context, as British analysts, we have been influenced mainly by the third, most limited group among object relations theories, the "English" (Kleinian) and "British" (Independent) schools, and we have tried to integrate them with some concepts of ego psychology (especially in the development of the concept of mentalization) and the empirically oriented psychoanalytic framework of attachment theory.

The early relationship with the caregiver emerged as a critical aspect of development from studies of severe character disorders by psycho-analysts in Britain. Fairbairn's (1952) focus on the individual's need for the other helped shift psychoanalytic attention from structure to con-tent, and profoundly influenced both British and North American psychoanalytic thinking. Building on this development, the self as a central part of the psychoanalytic model emerged in the work of Balint (1937, 1968) and Winnicott (1971). The concept of the caretaker or false self, as a defensive structure created to master trauma in a context of total dependency, has become an essential developmental construct. Winnicott's (1965) notions of primary maternal preoccupation, tran-sitional phenomena, the holding environment, and the mirroring function of the caregiver have become widely regarded as useful con-cepts in understanding the development of self-structure.

During the past half century the rise of object relations theories has been accompanied by a shift in psychoanalytic interest: there is a reduction of emphasis on the study of intrapsychic conflict, particu-larly conflicts relating to the sexual and aggressive drives, the central-ity of oedipal compromises, and the complementarity of biological and experiential forces in development (Lussier, 1988; Rangell, 1985; Spruiell, 1988). Instead psychoanalysis has moved increasingly towards an experientially based perspective, emphasizing the individual's experience of being with others and with the therapist in the transfer-ence (see, for example, Gill and Hoffman, 1982; Loewald, 1986; Schafer, 1983; Schwaber, 1983). This approach emphasizes phenomenological constructs such as individuals' experiences of themselves (see Stolorow et al., 1987) and of psychic as opposed to external reality (see McLaughlin, 1981; Michels, 1985). Patients in treatment commonly express them-selves in terms of relationships (Modell, 1990), and the move towards an object-relations-based metapsychology could be seen as led by an increasing cultural emphasis on the point of view of the subject, here the patient, and the therapist who learns from his subjective experience of the patient.

Object-relations theories vary along several dimensions. For exam-ple, while some move to replace drive theory approaches entirely (e.g. the interpersonal-relational schools, Mitchell and Black, 1995) others are built out of drive theory (e.g. Winnicott, 1962), while others derive drive theory from an object-relations approach (e.g. Kernberg, 1982). Object-relations theories also differ in their focus on mechanisms underlying personality functioning. For example, in general systems theory approaches, the mental mechanism underpinning internalized relationship representations is at the heart of the theory (e.g. Stern, 1985), whereas in self-psychology models object-relations are merely a route to a psychology of the self (e.g. Bacal, 1990).

Object-relations theories nevertheless share some assumptions. These include: (1) that severe pathology has pre-oedipal origins (i.e., the first 3 years of life); (2) that the pattern of relationships with objects becomes increasingly complex with development; (3) that the stages of this development follow a sequence across cultures, which may be distorted by personal trauma; (4) that early patterns of object-relations tend to be repeated through life; (5) that disturbances in these relations developmentally map onto pathology (see Westen, 1989); and (6) that transference provides a window on early relationship patterns. Friedman (1988) differentiates between "hard" and "soft" object-relations theories. Hard theories (including those of Klein, Fairbairn, and Kernberg) emphasize hate, envy, and destructiveness, and techniques confronting the unconsciously damaging impulses that result. Soft object-relations theorists (Balint, Winnicott, and Kohut) see the potential of love, innocence, growth, and creativity and empha-size techniques that allow progressive unfolding, with acceptance of regression and resistance.

Akhtar (1992) has usefully extended this contrast, using Strenger's (1989) model of the "classic" and "romantic" visions of man offered by psychoanalysts. The classic view would encompass the traditions of Melanie Klein, Kernberg, and some British object-relations theorists. The romantic approach perhaps originates with the work of Ferenczi and is well represented in the work of Balint, Winnicott, and Guntrip in the UK, and Modell and Adler in the United States. The first approach views psychopathology largely in terms of conflict; the second in terms of deficit. Acting out is seen as an inevitable conse-quence of deep-rooted pathology in the classic view, whilst the romantic view sees it as a manifestation of hope that the environment may reverse the damage done. There are approaches that combine the classic and the romantic. Kohut and Kernberg propose models of development that are pure representatives of neither tradition, and we would also see ourselves between the extremes.

Kernberg's contribution to the development of psychoanalytic thought deserves special mention as it has informed the way of formulating the focal problem we are following. Kernberg's systematic integration of structural theory and object-relations theory (Kernberg, 1976b, 1982, 1987) has been highly influential, particularly in relation to PDs. His model of psychopathology is developmental, in the sense that personality disturbance is seen to reflect the limited capacities of the young child to address intrapsychic conflict. Neurotic object-relations show much less defensive disintegration of the representation of self and objects into libidinally invested part-object-relations. In PD, part-object-relations are formed under the impact of diffuse, overwhelming emotional states—ecstatic or terrifying and painful ones—prompting persecutory relations between self and object.

Object-relations theories thus stand against Freud's assumption that psychic structure evolves intrapsychically whatever the child's relationships. Freud's suggestion that the mind is shaped by frustration of the child's drives allows for only one type of object-relationship (where the child's needs are frustrated) to play a part in the creation of mental structures and functions. Freudian and object-relations theory differ in the heterogeneity of possible relationship patterns seen in the latter as shaping mental structures. These theories assume that the child's mind is shaped by all early experiences with the caregiver, and our approach follows this assumption. Some theories, for example attachment theory, which we focus on below, assume an autonomous "relationship drive" which impels the infant into contact and preoccupation with the caregiver independent of the gratification of primary needs.

Ego functioning and theories of attachment

Child analysts (e.g. Fraiberg, 1969, 1980; Freud, 1965) helped us see that symptomatology is not a fixed formation, but rather a dynamic entity superimposed upon, and intertwined with, an underlying developmental process. Anna Freud's studies of children under great social stress led her to formulate a relatively comprehensive developmental theory, where the child's emotional and cognitive maturity could be mapped independently of diagnosable pathology. Her focus on the developmental processes (Freud, 1965) underlying ego capacities, and their relationship to psychological disturbance, is continued in the role of the capacity for mentalization in our framework.

Another important theorist in the background of our clinical application of attachment concepts here is Margaret Mahler, who drew attention to the paradox of self-development, that a separate identity implies the giving up of a highly gratifying closeness with the caregiver. Her observations of the "ambitendency" of children in their second year of life were helpful in understanding individuals with chronic problems of consolidating their individuality. Mahler's framework highlights the importance of the caregiver in facilitating separation. A traumatized, troubled parent may hinder rather than help a child's adaptation (Terr, 1983), and an abusive parent may altogether inhibit the process of social referencing (Cicchetti, 1990b; Hesse and Cicchetti, 1982). The pathogenic potential of the withdrawing object, when confronted with the child's wish for separateness, was further elaborated by Masten (1982) and Rinsley (1977), and is helpful in accounting for the transgenerational aspects of psychological disturbance.

Sandler's development of Anna Freud's and Edith Jacobson's work represents an early, inspired integration of the developmental perspective with psychoanalytic theory. At the core of Sandler's formulation lies the representational structure that contains both reality and distortion, and is the driving force of psychic life. A further important component of his model is the notion of the "background of safety" (Sandler, 1987), closely tied to Bowlby's concept of secure attachment and the secure base.

Bowlby's (1969, 1973, 1980) work on separation and loss strongly focused the attention of both clinicians and researchers on the importance of the security (safety, availability, and predictability) of the earliest relationships. His cognitive-systems model of the internalization of interpersonal relationships, that is, internal working models (IWMs), consistent with object-relations theory (Fairbairn, 1952; Kernberg, 1975) and elaborated by other attachment theorists (Bretherton, 1985; Crittenden, 1990; Main et al., 1985), has been particularly influential.

Along with the idea of the secure base, one of the most central concepts to attachment theory has been that of IWMs (Bowlby, 1973). Bowlby saw the attachment behavioral system as organized by a set of expectations built through experience. This idea has been creatively developed by several major contributors (e.g. Bretherton and Munholland, 1999; Crittenden, 1994; Main, 1991; Sroufe, 1996). Four representational systems are implied in these reformulations: (1) expectations of how caregivers will interact, beginning in the first year of life and later modified; (2) event representations in which general and specific memories of attachment-related experiences are stored; (3) autobiographical memories connected through personal meaning; and (4) understanding of one's own feelings and motives, and those of others.

This concept has had very broad application. Bowlby's developmental model highlights the transgenerational nature of IWMs: our view of ourselves depends upon the working model of relationships which characterized our caregivers. Empirical research has produced very robust findings (see van IJzendoorn, 1995); for example that an infant's security is well predicted from parental mental representations—coherence of narrative, and mentalization in relation to early experience—assessed before the birth of the child (e.g. Fonagy et al., 1991a, b).

Although Bowlby recognized (1973) that IWMs involved internal objects and object-relationships, he thought these were largely formed through external experience: "The varied expectations of the accessibility and responsiveness of attachment figures that different individuals develop during the years of immaturity are tolerably accurate reflections of the experiences those individuals have actually had" (Bowlby, 1973: 235). IWMs of the self and of parents are thus first built on early representations of the relationship, then evolve into freestanding yet interlocking images of the self and attachment figures (Bretherton, 1985). By interlocking, it is meant that a child who has IWMs of attachment figures as unloving and rejecting will in turn hold a model of the self as unlovable, unworthy, boring, etc. By contrast, a child who holds IWMs of attachment figures as loving and sensitive to their needs will hold a complementary model of the self as deserving their love and care.

Clearly, IWMs will only be adaptive for the person holding them if they enable that person to anticipate how people will behave towards them in future important situations (will loved ones protect them if they are sick, injured, in danger, or simply feeling bad, or will they not notice, not care, be cruel, or misunderstand?). Accurate anticipation requires that earlier experiences, on which prediction is based, have been perceived fairly realistically. Here, one immediately sees that distorted perceptions (e.g. by the operation of primitive defenses), and cognitive limitations natural at early stages of development, may lead a young child to draw wrong conclusions from half-understood interactions. If the underlying distortions are not corrected, they may be reinforced rather than modified in more realistic directions by later experiences. The protective value of IWMs could then be undermined and replaced by self-defeating misattributions and defensive strategies. These can be seen in the organized but "insecure" forms of attachment behavior and representation, described by attachment researchers and summarized later in this chapter, and familiar to psychotherapists.

Bowlby's development of attachment theory initially drew heated criticism from psychoanalysts (Fonagy, 2001). However, some features that made it anathema at first have gradually come to be seen as advantages: the introduction of biological principles in understanding personality and relationships—really a reintroduction because of course Freud began with that framework; a linking of empirical and theoretical evidence, and related to that, building bridges with a range of neighboring disciplines; and attention to the nonconscious (procedural or implicit) as well as dynamically unconscious determinants of our feelings, thoughts, and actions. These procedural or implicit determinants of personality structure and affect regulation are seen by us as closely relevant to the understanding of character development and PD, and to the mood disorders of many of our patients.

Finally, we should refer to the work of Stern, beginning with his 1985 book, a milestone in psychoanalytic theorization of development as reflected in the transference. His focus is the reorganization of subjective perspectives on self and other as these occur with the emergence of new maturational capacities. Stern deals with several qualitatively different senses of self, each developmentally anchored. He is perhaps closest to Sandler in his psychoanalytic model of the mind, but his formulation of object-relations also has much in common with those of Bowlby and Kernberg. Many of Stern's suggestions have proved to be highly valuable clinically, including his notion of an early core self and the role of the schema-of-being-with the other. These concepts, like those of Kernberg, can be seen to inform the integrative approach we propose in the current work.

Interpersonal psychoanalysis: the contribution of Harry Stack Sullivan

Sullivan is a neglected figure within contemporary psychoanalysis. An American psychiatrist working in the 1930s and 1940s, he was one of the main proponents of a particular strand of psychodynamic thinking called interpersonal psychiatry or interpersonal psychoanalysis which provided an alternative to Freud's drive theory. Although many of his ideas were shared by contemporaries, such by Eric Fromm and Karen Horney, Sullivan was a more fervent critic of Freud's emphasis on the importance of infantile sexuality and on intrapsychic conflict. By contrast, Sullivan emphasized the importance of external reality, for example, of the culture and society an individual grows up in, as well as of interconnectedness, which he understood to be central to understanding the development of an individual's personality and their difficulties.

Sullivan did not disregard the importance of intrapsychic experience, though he has been criticized for this, but it is true that in his writings, perhaps because he had to uphold a contrasting position, his primary emphasis is on the individual's current relationships and how these impact on evolving personality and psychopathology. Yet his notion of "personification" (i.e., the way a person comes to know the world through a set of internal assumptions/fantasies about the self and others based on developmental experience) is akin to the notion of an internal world. Moreover there are clear overlaps in his ideas with both attachment theory and object-relations theory, as we have seen, in light of his emphasis on the early mother–child relationship. Consistent with all psychoanalytic models, behavior and psychopathology were understood by Sullivan in relation to both historical and current interpersonal contexts.

In Sullivan's theory (1953) depression and anxiety are simply manifestations of the distortion and complexities of an individual's interpersonal relationships—a conceptualization that also informs DIT. In contemporary interpersonal models (see Kiesler, 1996) symptoms are seen to result primarily from problematic interactional patterns, which have become entrenched and can lead to extreme interpersonal behavior. This is simply another way of acknowledging the importance of internalized early interactional patterns, which become dominant and may significantly distort the individual's capacity to appraise what is happening in their relationship with others.

Sullivan's emphasis on actual (i.e., not fantasized) interpersonal exchanges, on how the patient communicates with the other person, and on the assumptions the patient makes about what the other person may be thinking or feeling are all very consistent with the focus in DIT on current relationships and functioning, including our emphasis on underlying attachment models and how mentalization in relation to external relationships is commonly distorted by these. The indirect, confusing, incongruous, and typically self-defeating communications that transpire in human relationships become the focus of intervention; this helps the patient identify their own contribution to recreating particular interpersonal scenarios, which are deeply distressing, but may nevertheless be perfectly understandable in light of developmental models that have become internalized. In particular, the relationship that develops between the patient and therapist provides a vehicle for helping the patient to understand some of the more automatic, unconscious assumptions they make about himself and others, and which can give rise to the onset of symptoms.

DIT also borrows from some of the technical principles that guided Sullivan's approach to the therapeutic situation itself. In particular Sullivan believed that humans strive to minimize insecurity. In his view, interpersonal behaviors, even ultimately self-defeating ones, could nevertheless be understood as attempts to avoid anxiety or depression or to establish/maintain self-esteem. Consequently, and of particular importance to Sullivan, was the psychotherapist's understanding and management of the patient's anxiety, present in the form of the patient's expectations and fear of the psychotherapist's disapproval and the interpersonal defenses that might be activated in order to avoid this experience of insecurity. As far as Sullivan was concerned, one of the psychotherapist's primary responsibilities was, as he put it, to "integrate the situation," that is, join with the patient to create an atmosphere of "interpersonal security."

Sullivan strongly favored an engaged, active therapeutic stance that tried to foster this sense of safety. He was very clear that interpersonal learning could only occur in a situation where the patient felt relatively safe, rather than in an atmosphere that was more likely to generate the patient's anxiety, such as being in a room with a relatively uncommunicative therapist. The stance that he therefore advocated was one that he terms "respectful seriousness." He believed that empathy was an interpersonal process worked out between the participants during the course of the therapy based on the patient's actual experience.

Along with all contemporary psychoanalytic models Sullivan understood that the patient's perceptions of the therapist were strongly shaped by the patient's experience prior to the treatment (that is, the transference brought to it). However, he emphasized that it was also shaped by the patient's actual experience during the therapy, and that careful attention needed to be paid to these perceptions. For Sullivan this needed to include therefore an understanding not only of the transference, but also of what he termed the "real" relationship with the therapist, including the impact of the psychotherapist's cultural role, anxieties, foibles, etc. In other words, Sullivan saw the therapeutic relationship as fundamentally intersubjective.

By paying careful attention to what transpired between the patient and the therapist the therapeutic situation was thus seen by Sullivan to provide an opportunity for "facilitating interpersonal learning." This is one of the core strategies of DIT.

Conclusions

The three sets of theories that we draw on and that we have briefly reviewed here reflect certain core assumptions that underpin DIT and its strategies (see Chapter 3). Most notably these include (a) the social origins and nature of individual subjectivity, (b) the importance of attachments as the building blocks of the mind, and as the context for developing crucial social cognitive capacities, (c) the impact of internalized, unconscious "self" and "other" representations on current interpersonal functioning, and (d) the importance of the capacity to mentalize experience without which the individual is more vulnerable to developmentally earlier modes of experiencing internal reality which, in turn, undermine the capacity to resolve interpersonal difficulties.

The following chapters will illustrate how these assumptions translate into technical recommendations and how they give shape to DIT's unifying therapeutic strategy, namely the identification of a specific interpersonal-affective focus (i.e., the IPAF).

Chapter 2

Why Dynamic Interpersonal Therapy for Mood Disorders?

The development of a protocol aimed at the treatment of a diagnostic entity such as depression or anxiety will be anathema to some psychodynamic practitioners. Traditionally symptoms and diagnosis have not held much currency within psychoanalytic thinking. In this chapter we will review some of the issues that invariably arise in this respect before outlining our psychodynamic framework for understanding mood disorders. We will conclude with a consideration of how to assess suitability for DIT.

Psychodynamic approaches and diagnostic classification

A controversial issue, which so far we have skirted around, concerns the status of psychiatric diagnosis and nosology. An approach primarily led by psychiatric formulation runs counter to the traditional psychoanalytic emphasis on the focus on the unconscious and the individual psychodynamics of every case. Our primary interest is typically *in whom* the depression or anxiety is occurring. In other words, we consider it vital in any treatment intervention to understand symptoms in the context of personality structure: for example, panic attacks in a narcissistic individual are lived out very differently than in a characterologically avoidant individual. The awareness of this context of the wider personality is inherent in DIT.

Psychiatric classification based on operational criteria, which first entered clinical practice via DSM-III (American Psychiatric Association, 1980), has many advantages, not least that it contributed to convincing decision-makers that psychiatric illness was measurable and predictable.

No one would claim that systems are any more than imperfect reflections of psychiatry's transition toward empiricism, objectification, and broadly based construction of new scientific theories. Yet nowadays we operate in an external world in which systems like DSM-IV (and shortly DSM-V) or ICD-10 give shape to how research is conducted, to the configuration of clinical services, and hence to how funding is prioritized.

When psychodynamic therapists engage with and use classification systems they do so as a concession to pragmatism (records, reporting, reimbursement, research, etc.), but experience the use of diagnostic categories as something with the potential to take the heart and soul out of psychotherapy. Many would probably prefer to diagnose patients as resembling prototypes, fictional characters such as Ophelia or Heathcliff, rather than use the sterile language of DSM or ICD.

Although objections to nosology are common, there is no shortage of examples of psychodynamic clinicians assigning individuals to categories such as narcissistic, masochistic, and even psychopathic. The tension appears to lie therefore not so much around whether "diagnosing" per se is helpful or not, but more around what system is used. There are indeed profound inconsistencies between a psychiatric diagnostic and a psychodynamic diagnostic approach, many of which are rooted in the respective history of the two disciplines. Psychoanalysts object to diagnostic systems, believing them to be regressions to a descriptive psychiatry redolent of the end of the nineteenth century and against which Freud rebelled by advancing a model of mental disorder based on hypothetical psychological mechanisms (e.g. the diagnosis of neurosis is based on the theories of drive, anxiety, and defense).

The difference between the two approaches to classification lies in the logic each one follows to arrive at their conclusions. As Drew Westen and Jonathan Shedler (2004) pointed out, the identification of a definitive list of symptoms and signs poorly fits psychodynamic clinical thinking (Shedler et al., 2010). The latter is based on categories drawing on emergent prototypes. Psychotherapists do not think of necessary and sufficient features in arriving at categorical decisions, but rather think of the typicality of an individual relative to an ideal type—perhaps never seen but based on the accumulation of clinical cases treated and studied.

Compared with the psychodynamic formulation and the decision about suitability for therapy, diagnosis has been relatively underemphasized in psychotherapy training programs. It is often claimed that a genuine understanding of an individual's pathology can only be made at the end of the therapy. By contrast, in modern medicine, the initial diagnosis represents the quintessence of competent practice and the necessary antecedent for rational choice of therapy.[1] Much of the evidence on the effectiveness of psychotherapy depends on psychiatric classification. Until recently funding for expensive RCTs depended on reliable and valid diagnostic conditions being established for participants.

Tom Insel, the director of the National Institute Mental Health (NIMH), anticipating the new edition of the DSM (DSM-V) laid out the expectation of the funding body in relation to a current approach to mental disorder. The NIMH Research Domain Criteria (RDoC) Project focuses on pathophysiology that will help identify new targets for treatment development, detect subgroups for treatment selection, and thus provide a better match between research findings and clinical decision making. RDoC classification rests on three assumptions: (1) mental disorders are disorders of brain circuits, (2) these can be identified with tools of neuroscience, and (3) data will yield biosignatures useful for clinical management. Strangely, this approach is closer to the mechanism-oriented approach that Freud pioneered, although the mechanisms RDoC points to are not psychological but physiological.

Unless we adopt a dualist stance, we should feel confident that a reliable and robust psychological mechanism-based system, which is valuable in establishing suitability for treatment, will also correspond to key brain processes relevant to neuroscience. This is certainly true for two constructs of relevance to DIT: attachment (Insel, 2003; Strathearn et al., 2009) and mentalization (Frith and Frith, 2006; Van Overwalle, 2009), and is the case for other features of depression and anxiety, for example, memory deficits (Whalley et al., 2009).

---

[1] Nor was psychoanalysis always opposed to diagnostic labels. Classically, Ernest Jones (1927) called for psychotherapists to be trained to distinguish OCD from bipolar illness, paranoid psychotic conditions from phobic disorders, and dysthimia from somatic conditions (p. 183).

Where does DIT situate itself in these debates? The descriptive approach to diagnosis implicitly taken by us in this book need not alarm practitioners: it is taken primarily for pragmatic reasons. We recognize that most formal outcome research and some treatment services are organized according to diagnostic categories, hence we favor an approach to bridging these very different frameworks at a pragmatic level.

The diagnosis of major depressive or anxiety disorder (MDD), in our view, constitutes only one (small) part of a complete formulation and treatment plan. A judgment about the contribution of interacting psychological, biological, and social systems to the patient's descriptive presentation is a necessary addition to an ICD or DSM diagnosis. The descriptive and psychodynamic approaches to formulation, such as the ones we adopt (with a rather broad brush) in DIT, are not inherently opposed; rather, they are overlapping, complementary, and necessary to each other. We assume, and recommend, an integrated approach where clinicians adopt a research diagnostic and a psychodynamic approach to formulation.

Mood disorders: depression and anxiety

"Depression," a patient said, "feels like wearing a beautifully embroidered black veil. I know I can't see things clearly through it, but I don't know that I could reveal myself to the world without it." This comment captures vividly the complexity of depression: it is a disabling condition and yet the relationship an individual may have with it—that is, its function in the patient's psychic economy—may make the patient fearful of change and hence resistant to being helped. Other patients with both depression and anxiety commonly use metaphors of feeling weighed down, trapped, or deadened to convey the sense of threat and dread which both conditions tend to bring with them.

The great majority of our mood-disordered patients presenting for psychotherapy in outpatient and primary care settings are troubled by symptoms of both depression and anxiety disorders. In addition they may have various other diagnosable symptoms, which have sometimes developed alongside the mood disturbance. Examples would be disturbances of eating, abuse of other substances (perhaps originally for self-medication), and patterns of dependence, misery, self-harm, or avoidance which may have become so chronic as to fulfil criteria for a chronic disorder such as dysthymia or a PD.

In DIT we take the view that patients across the spectrum of mood disorders, with varying combinations of diagnostic labels, have in common a tendency to organize social experiences according to underlying unconscious expectations of self and other that trigger particular affects. Once active in the mind such (typically unconscious) interpersonal configurations lead to mental and behavioral defensive strategies, which are in turn maladaptive. We apply the structure of focusing on an IPAF across the spectrum, as long as there is not an alternative treatment approach that is needed more immediately (e.g. detoxification, management of suicidal behavior, or treatment of agoraphobia which would prevent the person from getting to sessions).

Below, we give some background to by far the two most commonly presenting types of disorder in this range, depression and anxiety, which frequently go together in primary care and outpatient settings. The DIT therapist needs to be conscious that both of these painful states of mind are likely to be consequences of the conflictual unconscious "script" represented by the IPAF, and that both need to be much improved if the patient is to become well enough to maintain their progress after therapy ends.

Depression is a common and often complex condition that typically manifests early in life: 40 percent of depressed people experienced a first episode by age 20 (Eaton et al., 2008). It interferes with social and occupational functioning, is associated with considerable morbidity, and carries a significant risk of mortality through suicide (Ustun et al., 2004). Incomplete recovery and relapse are all too common. Following the first episode of major depression, people often go on to have at least one more episode (Kupfer, 1991) and the risk of further relapse rises sharply to 70 and 90 percent after the second and third episodes respectively (Kupfer, 1991). Anxiety disorders are also prevalent, especially social anxiety and phobias, and these, like depression, tend to begin in childhood (Blackmore et al., 2009). GAD tends to start later but to be more chronic (Yonkers et al., 1996).

The aetiology of depression and anxiety is not fully understood, but is likely to be overdetermined by psychological, social, and biological processes (Fonagy, 2010; Goldberg, 2010; Malhi et al., 2009; Suarez et al., 2008; Taylor, 2010). It has also been shown to be common, as stated above, for depressed people to have a comorbid psychiatric diagnosis (e.g. anxiety, alcohol abuse, various PDs) (Kessler et al., 1996; Moffitt et al., 2007). Importantly in considering the approach in DIT, it has been shown that where patients present with depression and comorbid anxiety disorders, the anxiety usually preceded the depression, and may therefore be an underlying focus of mood disturbance (Kessler et al., 1996). Patients meeting criteria for a MDD are nine times more likely than chance to meet criteria for other conditions (Angst and Dobler-Mikola, 1985). Similarly diagnosable anxiety disorders commonly present with comorbid conditions, particularly depression; for example, a study of 279 patients with GAD found that 67 percent met criteria for MDD. Overall, 50–90 percent of patients with Axis I conditions also meet criteria for other Axis I or Axis II conditions (Westen et al., 2004).

Alongside the evident complexity of depression and anxiety, an apparently simplistic approach has prevailed at the level of service provision within the public health sector where the current emphasis on evidence-based practice has privileged CBT as the treatment of choice for both disorders. This "one size fits all" approach to treatment has strongly marginalized psychoanalytic interventions. The superiority of CBT in this respect has been rightly questioned, not because it is not helpful to many depressed and anxious patients, as it evidently is, but because it is not helpful to *all* such patients. RCTs show that, as with all available treatments, a substantial minority of patients do not benefit sufficiently—around 50 percent responding adequately across treatments, with half of those losing gains over the following year (e.g. Roth and Fonagy, 2005). No single treatment is the answer for everybody and a variety of approaches with some evidence of effectiveness should continue to be available.

Several publications have focused on the effectiveness of psychoanalytic approaches for depressed and anxious patients and have criticized the hegemony of CBT in this respect (Gabbard, Gunderson and Fonagy, 2004; Leichsenring et al., 2004). Even so, the all too frequent conflation of an underdeveloped evidence base for psychoanalytic interventions with a "weak" treatment prevails in the minds of those commissioning services. We will not rehearse these tensions here.

DIT formulates the presenting symptoms of mood disorders as responses to interpersonal difficulties/perceived threats to attachments (loss/separation) and hence also as threats to the self. It conceptualizes depression and anxiety with low mood in terms of an underlying temporary disorganization of the attachment system caused by current relationship problems, which in turn generates a range of distortions in thinking and feelings typical of chronically depressed and anxious states of mind. In the therapy a focus is maintained on this emotional "crisis" through an elaboration of the thoughts and feelings (conscious and unconscious) most characteristic of the particular patient, and relevant to his[2] depressed and anxious mood, as these emerge in the context of the therapeutic relationship. Through the focused exploration of the transference relationship the patient is helped to develop a better understanding of his subjective reactions to threats. Making implicit anxieties and concerns explicit through improving the patient's ability to reflect on his own and other's thoughts and feelings, in turn, enhances the patients' ability to cope with current attachment-related interpersonal threats and challenges.

DIT's starting point is rooted in the common clinical observation that patients who present as depressed and/or anxious almost invariably also present with difficulties and distress about their relationships. Although the patient may well experience his problem as "I cannot sleep and concentrate" or "I can't face going into crowded places, or going to work" the DIT therapist reframes such symptoms of anxiety and depression as manifestations of a relational disturbance, which the patient cannot understand, or understands in a maladaptive way, attributing to himself and others motivations which are unlikely or unhelpful. Once the patient is helped to make some changes in the

---

[2] For clarity and economy, the patient will be referred to as "he" and the therapist as "she."

way he approaches his relationship difficulties, depressive and anxious symptoms are typically alleviated.

There are many features of mood disorders that suggest that a dynamically oriented approach focusing on interpersonal issues is likely to be effective in addressing the symptoms. Interpersonal problems are marked in severe depression and anxiety disorders, and evident even in mild or moderate conditions (Luyten et al., 2005). This seems to be driven not only by the potential of persistent, irrationally depressed and anxious mood to elicit negative responses from others, but also by the inclination of depressed and anxious people to seek and generate interpersonal scenarios with the propensity to evoke distress, such as conflict or resistance to efforts to help, leading to social exclusion and rejection (see, e.g., Kiesler, 1983; Lewinsohn et al., 1980).

The recent work of psychoanalytic researchers Sidney Blatt and Patrick Luyten demonstrates that not only is vulnerability to depression associated with the unconscious generation of interpersonal stress, but also interpersonal factors explain much current data on the outcomes of treatments of depression (Blatt et al., 2010; Luyten et al., 2006). There is increasing agreement in the field that the interpersonal aspects of depression should be given comparable weight to the normally highlighted intrapersonal dimensions (e.g. Hammen, 2005). Similarly, the model of "triple vulnerability" to anxiety disorders posits—in addition to a biological substrate—factors of "generalized psychological vulnerability" such as experiences of negative parenting and a sense of uncontrollability, coupled with "specific psychological vulnerability," especially interpersonal triggering events such as loss of a loved one, relationship difficulties, and trauma such as assault (Suarez et al., 2008).

While the literature on distorted information-processing in depression and anxiety disorders largely speaks to distortions of conscious cognition (Beck et al., 1979; Clark and Wells, 1995; Kyte and Goodyer, 2008), some concepts in this literature, such as the dominance of a hopeless, helpless attributional style (Abramson et al., 1978), echo classical psychoanalytic writings which link these observations to unconscious projective and introjective processes (Engel and Schmale, 1967).

DIT as an approach includes attention to apparent dysfunctions in interpersonal cognition concerned with an individual's distorted and inadequate understanding of others' thoughts and feelings (that is, mentalization). The consideration of mentalization within DIT, including the use of mentalization techniques to introduce different perspectives on the selected IPAF, is consistent with recently accumulating data demonstrating theory of mind deficits in patients with unipolar and bipolar depressive disorders (Inoue et al., 2004, 2006; Kerr et al., 2003; Lee et al., 2005; Montag et al., 2010).

Measures of mentalizing in the attachment context also yield indications of a deficit associated with depression (Fischer-Kern et al., 2008; Fonagy et al., 1996; Müller et al., 2006). This is important as DIT assumes failures of self and other understanding in depression to be strongly tied to particular self–other interaction patterns evolved from childhood experiences, real or fantasized (see Chapter 5, The Interpersonal-Affective Focus). Patients with anxiety disorders who are not significantly depressed may have less difficulty with mentalization; their work on the IPAF may be less interfered with by a conviction that their perception of people's motives is the only one possible.

DIT has a dual focus on interpersonal and affective issues. The affective issues of greatest relevance center on attachment-related concerns. Insecurely attached individuals are more likely to have more frequent anxiety states (with a high background level of chronic anxiety) and depressive episodes, residual symptoms, use more pharmacotherapy, and are more likely to be impaired in their social functioning (Conradi and de Jonge, 2009).

There is a substantial body of work linking vulnerability to depression to insecure attachment (Bifulco et al., 2002a, b; Lee and Hankin, 2009). Blatt's theory of depression identifies two classes of attachment history-based cognitive-affective schemata most likely to be found in depression: interpersonal dependency and excessive self-criticism (Blatt, 2008; Blatt and Luyten, 2009) linked to preoccupied and avoidant patterns of attachment respectively (Blatt and Luyten, 2009). There has also been extensive research on parent–child attachment and the development of anxiety disorders (see Chorpita and Barlow, 1998). Much of this has focused on parental overprotection, separation anxiety, and the child's increasing fear of loss of control (Silove et al., 1991), with intolerance of uncertainty which becomes interpersonally stressful as the child needs to function out-side the home.

For decades, evidence has been accumulating linking childhood adversity, likely to disrupt attachment, to adult vulnerability for depression (Brown and Harris, 1978, 1989) and anxiety (Torgerson, 1986). The association is increasingly well understood in terms of the effects of attachment experiences on the stress system (Heim et al., 2008) and the moderation of the impact of later stressful experiences by acquiring a secure state of mind in relation to attachment history (Bakermans-Kranenburg et al., 2008).

Attachment experiences also link mentalizing and depression (Heim et al., 2008; Luyten et al., 2009). A reduced capacity to think about mental states may be related to personal histories (e.g. trauma) but may also be a secondary consequence of disordered mood (Luyten et al., 2011). Indications of a failure of mentalizing are not hard to find. There is a reemergence of a pre-reflective, physical self-experience in place of a psychological self-experience (Fonagy and Target, 2000). Psychological experience is felt to be far too real, with a common equation between psychological and physical pain and emotional and physical exhaustion (Van Houdenhove and Luyten, 2009). A state of "hyperembodiment" ensues, in which subjective experiences are primarily felt to be physical in nature. Worries can feel like genuine weights on one's shoulders, and the criticism of others threatens the sense of integrity of the embodied self. The therapeutic task is to help the patient elaborate the state of mind that is experienced as a physical symptom rather than being available for consideration and reappraisal as a belief or a thought. The lack of drive, which is at the heart of depression, is similarly seen as a regressive embodiment of disempowering thought.

Similarly, the intensity of worries about the future, and the over-powering nature of self-blame associated with past experience, imply an underlying loss of symbolic perspective, where thought gains inappropriate, concrete strength by being awarded the same status as physical reality. In the absence of a capacity to reflect on experience, self-questioning turns into an irresolvable and interminable persecutory attack upon the self-representation.

In the formulation of depression and anxiety advanced in support of DIT, distortions of cognitions are considered to indicate varying failures of mentalization, which may be concrete thinking, or indications of pseudo-mentalizing (also referred to as "hypermentalizing"). In the latter case, the patient's description of the mental states of others or his own mental state reflects an apparent thoughtfulness, but this lacks some essential features of genuine mentalization; it is a partial understanding, containing some truth, but is excessively detailed and often repetitive. Characteristics include a sense of certainty about mental states, including the unrealistic assumption that one can directly know someone else's mind, and limiting what is attributed to the other's mental state to ideas and themes that reinforce the individual's existing perspective which, however painful and self-destructive, is held on to for powerful unconscious reasons.

A genuine capacity to reflect on one's own experience should thus not be confused with hypermentalization, nor with rumination. Whereas rumination leads to exacerbations of depressive and anxious cognitions, effective self-reflection normally leads to lifting of negative moods (Allen et al., 2008). This assumption is borne out by studies showing a distinction between reflection and brooding, with the former being related to improved mood, the latter with greater depression and suicidal ideation.

Assessing suitability for DIT

If there is an art to psychotherapy then surely this is most relevant to the assessment for suitability because we are short on science in this domain. Despite the considerable advances we have made in understanding many aspects of the therapeutic process and its outcomes across a range of psychological therapies, our capacity to reliably assess "what works for whom" remains limited. When it comes to the assessment of suitability a core competence is indeed the ability to draw on knowledge that pre-therapy patient characteristics are *not* significantly predictive of outcome for psychodynamic therapy, whatever its particular "brand" (Lemma et al., 2008).

Notwithstanding this cautionary note, it would be impossible to make any decisions if we were not informed at least by the wealth of practice-based evidence that provides some markers for assessing suitability for a psychodynamic approach. Certain dimensions of the patient's experience (intrapsychic, interpersonal, and pragmatic) are

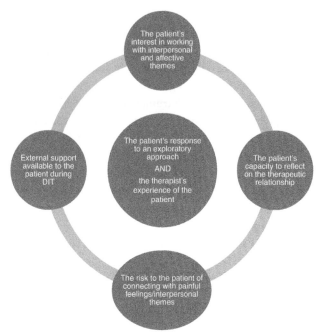

Figure 2.1 Dimensions to be explored when assessing suitability.

pertinent to assessing when DIT may or may not be indicated for some patients, as well as to how it may need to be adapted to meet the patient's needs. Each of the following domains thus provides a *partial* vantage point from which to consider DIT's suitability. Considered together they amount to guidelines for assessing suitability rather than evidence-based recommendations (see Figure 2.1).

The patient's response to an exploratory approach

The DIT therapist aims to engage the patient in a process of reflection on his states of mind in the context of relationships, including the therapeutic one: hence it makes different demands on the patient relative to, say, CBT or IPT. Moreover, despite the greater therapist activity given the time-limited nature of the therapy, there is still a *relative* lack of therapist direction compared to other therapies. The therapist approaches the therapeutic situation with an analytic attitude so as to observe the patient's interaction with her and evaluate what adaptations may be necessary to support the patient's capacity to work within an analytic frame. This takes us back to the fundamental importance of adopting a flexible approach that prioritizes meeting the patient where he is at rather than trying, at all costs, to fit him into a model that is not responsive to his needs.

Having said this, because the DIT therapist adopts an analytic stance this makes particular demands on the patient, which may render it unsuitable and/or uncongenial for some. An important indicator of suitability is therefore the assessment of how the patient manages without systematic therapist-imposed direction in the session (e.g. do they become anxious or paranoid?) and the extent to which the patient is responsive to the invitation to reflect on what is happening in his life as opposed to primarily seeking relief from symptoms through practical strategies.

The patient's interest in working with interpersonal and affective themes

Every patient comes to an assessment with his own language and frame of reference for emotional distress, with his own theories consonant with cultural idioms for the expression of emotional distress. Often the assessment provides an opportunity for sharing different narratives about the problem. The patient may find that DIT's interpersonal and affective emphasis is meaningful and helpful and he may thus shift, say, from his former biochemical explanation to a more psychological one. This is not always the case, however. It is therefore important to listen out for whether the patient's own narrative maps onto the DIT one. We are looking for some compatibility between treatment rationale and the patient's own theories. There is little point in offering DIT to a patient who is convinced his problems are related to a genetic predisposition or who believes that it is all down to his faulty thinking. The aim of assessment is not to work towards getting the patient to take on our point of view but to find a good-enough fit between our knowledge of the patient's difficulties and the therapeutic approach most congenial to the patient's own way of thinking, or philosophy of life, that could best address those difficulties.

DIT is unequivocally focused on the patient's interpersonal functioning in his current life and in the therapeutic interaction, and on his emotional experience. Given this focus, it is essential to gauge early on the patient's interest in working with these themes. This requires the therapist to engage the patient's interest in DIT by making a trial interpretation (see Chapter 5) that connects the patient's presenting difficulties/feelings/symptoms to their past and current relationships and behavior.

Capacity to reflect on the therapeutic relationship

We hope that our patients will be able to develop an emotionally "live" relationship with us. It will arouse a host of feelings—positive and negative—some of which may feel terrifying. The patient's grip on reality, and hence his appreciation of the "as if" quality of the transference, is therefore a vital prerequisite. In order for the patient to use and benefit from DIT it is important that he can be helped to reflect on the therapeutic relationship whilst maintaining reality testing. When this capacity is absent the patient no longer experiences us, for example, *as if* we were an abusive parent; rather, in his experience we *are* the abusive parent. A symbol is experienced as representing an object. When the symbol and the thing it symbolizes cannot be distinguished this reflects a breakdown in symbolic functioning which is psychically devastating and a contraindication for DIT.

One of the most meaningful indicators of suitability is the patient's response to the therapist's attempts to understand him, for example, does the patient feel relieved or persecuted by the therapist's focus on his mind or on what may be happening between them in therapy. Interpretations that draw the patient's attention to his unconscious experience of the therapy (e.g. about how the patient may be feeling anxious about the prospect of this kind of engagement) are especially helpful. The patient's response will help the therapist to develop a picture of the patient's readiness and motivation at this point in time to engage with the affective and interpersonal focus of the therapy, and more specifically to determine the extent to which the patient can:

◆ stand back from his experience and observe his own mind

◆ receive and make use of what we can offer

◆ work to a focus.

The patient's curiosity about his role in his difficulties

The DIT therapist is more explicitly supportive than might be the case in other dynamic models, but she is nevertheless also challenging because of DIT's emphasis on supporting the patient to make some actual changes in how he relates to others. It is never long before the patient realizes, for example, that his narrative about victimization will be gradually challenged by the therapist in order to invite him to reflect on his part in the repetitive pattern that has been selected as the focus of the therapy. This requires considerable motivation on the patient's part, especially when symptoms are ego-syntonic (i.e., they do not generate conflict).

How one assesses motivation is nevertheless complicated since it is a complex, multidimensional concept. There is, in fact, little agreement over the term. It is sometimes defined so broadly that it becomes synonymous with suitability for psychodynamic therapy (Truant, 1999). Clinical work makes one thing very clear, however: motivation does not refer to a static state of mind. Patients will traverse periods in therapy when their motivation is high and at other times the secondary gains from illness gain the upper hand and motivation wanes. The relative predominance of a motivation to change over unconscious gratification from the symptoms, which acts as a resistance to change, is an important factor to assess.

The assessment of motivation is of necessity inferential. It can be gleaned from a thorough exploration of the patient's previous experience of therapy, where applicable, and of his expectations of the new treatment. To assess motivation it may be helpful to explore the following areas with the patient:

- What is the patient's relationship to help? What did the patient find difficult or helpful in his former therapy, if anything? How realistic are his expectations of therapy? What difficulties does he envisage in relation to the treatment you are proposing to him? Does he display an active or passive stance? Is he hoping to be "cured" or does he give some indication that he appreciates that therapy will make demands on him and is not just down to the therapist?

◆ Is the patient's relationship to the therapist an overly idealized one? Some positive investment in the person of the therapist and her capacity to relieve suffering is necessary for a working alliance to be established, but this is quite different from the patient who takes a back seat and is expecting a magical transformation at the hands of an all-powerful therapist. Rigid idealization or denigration of a previous therapist should sound alarm bells and can be a poor prognostic sign.

◆ Is the patient motivated internally or by external sources? This question is typically related to the "why now" question. It is important to explore this because those who enter therapy at the behest of partners or other mental health professionals may establish a weaker alliance or misalliances that can undermine the treatment process. Generally speaking, the patient is motivated to work in therapy if he experiences his problems/symptoms at least to a degree as ego-dystonic. It is important here to distinguish between motivation for self-understanding (e.g. "I want to understand why I always end up feeling humiliated") and a search for concrete relief from symptoms or particular life situations (e.g. "I want to get out of the council estate I am in, that's getting me down"). Although in both cases the patient will be motivated to get some form of help it is unlikely that the second patient will find DIT congenial.

The risk to the patient of connecting with painful feelings/interpersonal themes, which could be difficult for them to manage (e.g. increasing risk to themselves), is balanced against the benefits of exploring issues in therapy.

Although the DIT therapist is encouraged to adopt a more supportive stance than is characteristic of some psychodynamic models, the therapy nevertheless does address unconscious conflict and defenses. It is important to assess the risk that this exploratory emphasis might expose the patient to. A key task in the assessment is therefore to realistically consider, with the patient, his capacity to work within a time-limited analytic frame. This requires some knowledge and formulation in the following domains:

◆ Knowledge of the patient's history of self-harm, violence, neglect, or self-defeating behaviors.

◆ Assessment of the patient's ego strength. This involves identifying whether the patient's difficulties restrict his self-observational capacity and other executive ego functions, which would contribute to diffuse boundaries and encourage acting out. A patient's ego strength is inferred from presentation at assessment. It reflects those personality assets that will enable the patient to overcome anxieties and acquire more adaptive defenses. At its most basic, ego strength refers to the patient's capacity to be in touch with reality whereby perception, thinking, and judgment are unimpaired. Ego strength reflects the patient's capacity to hold on to his identity in the face of psychic pain, without resorting to excessive distortion or denial. Ego weakness manifests itself in poor frustration tolerance and impulse control, a lack of tolerance of anxiety, and an absence of sublimatory activity. For example, a patient who is angry and has weak ego strength is less likely to be able to reflect on the source and meaning of his anger and may instead act on it and attack another person. The patient with more ego strength will either be able to think about his anger or might manage to sublimate it and channel it into some other more constructive activity, for example, exercise.

◆ The patient's capacity to persist with relationships and occupational or vocational endeavors in the face of challenges provides us with another opportunity to indirectly assess ego strength. This is why it is important to take an educational and occupational history: patients who present with histories of dropping out of education, being fired from jobs, or flitting from job to job would raise the question of whether they have a sufficiently well-developed capacity to persevere with stressful situations.

The external resources that could support the patient during the course of DIT

It is important here to keep in mind that we are not assessing whether the patient fits the model but rather the extent to which the model, and the context in which it is provided, can be adapted to meet the needs of the patient. A central feature of the assessment for DIT therefore involves an ability to identify and take account of external resources available to the patient and to the therapist when planning the intervention, such that due consideration is given to the need for additional supports through exploring the patient's external resources (e.g. sources of support, stability of housing, etc.) and the appropriateness of the setting in which the therapy will be offered relative to the patient's needs (e.g. for additional support from other professionals).

The therapist's experience with the patient in the session

All the dimensions we have outlined so far will give us important clues as to how the patient is likely to respond to DIT. However, the therapist's direct experience of being in the room with the patient is probably the most informative of all. Patients who "on paper" would seem unlikely candidates for DIT may nevertheless convey in their interaction in the room a glimmer of hope that with careful pacing by the therapist and adequate support both within and outside of the therapy, for example, they could make use of DIT. Here it is worth also noting that because of the more explicit supportive stance adopted by the DIT therapist, and its relatively more structured format, DIT may provide a useful bridge into longer-term psychodynamic therapy for patients who are not yet ready to avail themselves of this kind of intervention.

The therapist's appraisal of what the patient can tolerate and make use of is also gleaned from the therapist's reflection on the emotional impact the patient's presentation has on them (i.e., her countertransference). This rests on our ability to appraise the potential significance of our responses to understanding the patient's interpersonal patterns.

As will be apparent from the above list, when assessing suitability for DIT we will need to appraise several dimensions of the patient's experience, and of his context, and pool them together in order to take a view. As we will repeatedly emphasize throughout this book, a flexible approach is critically important in so far as some patients might at first struggle with some of the demands DIT may make on them, but a therapist capable of carefully titrating her interventions could well make it possible nonetheless for the patient to make use of DIT.

Chapter 3

Core Features and Strategies

The techniques used in DIT, which we will outline in detail in Chapter 7, are by no means exclusive to this approach, and will be familiar to psychodynamically trained clinicians. DIT, however, distinguishes itself at the level of its overall strategy because it is a time-limited therapy consisting of sixteen weekly sessions structured around the formulation and working through of a problematic, recurrent interpersonal-affective pattern that becomes the focus (the IPAF) (see Box 3.1).

DIT can be conceptualized as having three phases, each with distinctive aims and strategies. In this chapter we will give an overview of these three phases so as to sketch out the trajectory for the therapy. In subsequent chapters we will then go into the detail for each phase.

Aims

DIT has been developed to meet the needs of patients who are depressed and/or anxious. It primarily targets the patient's interpersonal functioning and the capacity to think about, and understand, changes in mood triggered by the activation in the mind of a particular self–other representation as the medium through which to reduce symptoms of depression and/or anxiety.

DIT thus has two primary aims:

1. To help the patient understand the connection between his presenting symptoms and what is happening in his relationships through identifying a core, unconscious, repetitive pattern of relating that becomes the focus of the therapy.

2. To encourage the patient's capacity to reflect on his own states of mind and so enhance his ability to manage interpersonal difficulties.

It is important to keep in mind DIT's dual aims because this will provide an orienting internal frame of reference for the therapist, which is especially helpful during the middle phase of the therapy when the therapist may struggle to stay focused (see Chapter 6).

Trajectory of the therapy

We conceptualize DIT as consisting of three phases. Many brief psychodynamic models also structure the therapy in a similar way: an *initial phase* concerned primarily with engaging the patient and assessing his difficulties, a *middle phase* during which the therapist focuses on an identified problem or pattern, and an *ending phase*, which reviews the progress made and helps the patient to say goodbye by focusing on the conscious and unconscious meaning for the patient of the separation from the therapist.

The three phases in DIT and their related aims and strategies are somewhat artificially divided and "timed" for the sake of descriptive clarity. In practice we would expect there to be significant flexibility in how and when the various strategies linked to each phase are implemented. For example, although we suggest that the formulation is shared with the patient at session 4, this may well only be possible in later sessions, and very occasionally a little sooner.

The initial phase (sessions 1–4)

Broadly speaking the first four sessions are devoted to the assessment of the problem and its dynamic formulation—what we refer to as the IPAF—and to engaging the patient through working in an explicitly collaborative way, involving him in refining the formulation (see Table 3.1).

This initial phase is fundamental to the subsequent course of DIT since the remainder of the therapy is structured around the exploration of the specific IPAF that emerges from this assessment. In our experience this is the phase that clinicians new to DIT find the most challenging, but also the most helpful since the practice of explicitly formulating a focus then provides an invaluable compass for the therapist's interventions during the subsequent two phases.

The middle phase (sessions 5–12)

The primary aim during this phase is simple: to intervene, using a range of techniques (see Chapter 7), so as to facilitate working through of the

Table 3.1 Initial phase: sessions 1–4

Aims:

♦ Engagement

♦ Exploration of depressive/anxiety symptoms (including risk factors) with an emphasis on the origins and psychological meaning of the symptoms

♦ Identification of strengths/resources in the patient and in their wider interpersonal network

♦ Formulation of focal area of work

Strategies:

♦ Identify patient's "interpersonal map" which includes a detailed picture of the patient's significant relationships and their connection with presenting problems

♦ Use attachment self-descriptions to characterize basic attachment style

♦ Focus on interpersonal circumstances and significant life events preceding onset of depression/anxiety and modulators of mood and/or anxiety

♦ Assessment of patient's current and past interpersonal functioning to identify recurring interpersonal pattern(s) that inform the patient's experience of his relationships

♦ Discuss and agree with the patient the formulation, treatment rationale, and goals

mutually agreed IPAF (see Table 3.2). The therapist's unwavering attention to the IPAF and to unpacking it, as it were, by helping the patient to consider its contribution to maintaining the problem/symptom(s) he is experiencing, its function in the patient's mind (including what it defends against), and its "cost" (i.e., the impact it has on his relationships, on his symptoms, etc.), is the central therapeutic strategy.

Sessions during this phase, in common with other psychodynamic approaches, share a more emergent quality to allow space for the elaboration of the patient's affective experience and of his imaginative life. Having said this, relative to longer-term psychodynamic models, the therapist is more active, inviting the patient, where possible, to gradually try out different ways of approaching interpersonal difficulties.

The ending phase (sessions 13–16)

Given DIT's focus on the importance of attachments, the meaning of the loss of the relationship with the therapist is singled out for exploration

Table 3.2 Middle phase: sessions 5–12

Aims:

♦ Working through of mutually agreed, interpersonal focal area

Strategies:

♦ Help patient to stay focused on the exploration of narratives about relationships (real or imagined)

♦ Keep focus on the patient's state of mind, not his behavior (link interpersonal processes with patient's mental states)

♦ Help patient to discover what he currently feels and how this relates to current and past interpersonal experiences, including in the relationship with the therapist

♦ Help patient to make connections between symptoms and interpersonal events

♦ Active, supportive stance to encourage the patient to try out new ways of resolving his difficulties (e.g. trying out new ways of communicating with others)

in the final sessions (see Table 3.3). Endings can mobilize particular feelings and fantasies very powerfully and the therapist is tasked with helping the patient to make sense of his experience of ending. Often the IPAF that has been worked on is relevant to understanding the patient's idiosyncratic experience of separation.

Alongside the exploration of the experience of ending, the therapist also uses the last few sessions as an opportunity to engage the patient in reviewing the work over the IPAF (which includes writing a "goodbye

Table 3.3 Ending phase: sessions 13–16

Aims

♦ To enable the patient to explore conflicts concerning loss, separation, and independence triggered by anticipated separation from the therapist

♦ To take stock of what has been achieved and plan for the future

Strategies

♦ Facilitate expression of patient's anxieties and fantasies about ending

♦ Review work that has been accomplished

♦ Acknowledge progress made

♦ Anticipate future difficulties/areas of vulnerability

♦ Write "goodbye" letter summarizing the work

letter" to the patient summarizing the IPAF), and consolidating the gains made as well as anticipating future vulnerabilities.

Our experience of training and supervising clinicians offering DIT suggests that this phased protocol enables dynamically oriented clinicians to achieve good results. Drawing on their established experience of working psychodynamically, the therapists structure their interventions guided by five relatively simple strategic steps in the course of a brief therapeutic engagement (Lemma et al., 2010):

1. Identify an attachment-related problem with a specific relational emotional focus that is felt by the patient to be currently making him feel depressed and/or anxious.

2. Work with the patient collaboratively to create an increasingly mentalistic picture of interpersonal issues raised by the problem.

3. Encourage the patient to explore the possibility of alternative ways of feeling and thinking ("playing with a new internal and external reality"), actively using the transference relationship to bring to the fore the patient's characteristic ways of relating.

4. Ensure the therapeutic process (of change in self) is reflected on.

Box 3.1 Core features of DIT

- Works on a circumscribed interpersonal and affective focus (IPAF)
- Focuses on the patient's mind rather than his behavior
- Time-limited (16 sessions)
- The therapeutic relationship is addressed and used to help the patient to explore the IPAF
- Makes use of expressive, supportive, mentalizing and, when appropriate, directive techniques to maximize change within a brief format
- Primarily targets enhanced interpersonal functioning and capacity for understanding self and other, rather than characterological change

5. Near the end of treatment present the patient with a written summary of the collaboratively created view of the person and the selected area of unconscious conflict, for him to hold on to, to reduce the risk of relapse.

In later chapters we will describe these strategies in more detail, but for now we will focus in broader terms on the three foci that are central to DIT and on the therapeutic stance characteristic of DIT.

The DIT foci

The interpersonal-affective focus

DIT adopts an idiographic approach to formulation. The primary task of the initial phase, which organizes DIT's therapeutic thrust, is to identify typically one dominant and recurring unconscious interpersonal pattern: the IPAF (see Chapter 5). This pattern is nested within an unconscious approach to attachment, dependence, and possible intimacy, which is captured by a broad description of the patient's dominant attachment style. The specific pattern then agreed as a focus for work with the patient is underpinned by a particular representation of self-in-relation-to-an-other that characterizes the patient's interpersonal style and that leads to difficulties in his relationships because it organizes interpersonal behavior. These representations are typically linked to a particular affect(s). Affects are understood to be responses to the activation, in the patients' mind, of a specific self–other representation (Kernberg, 1985).

Past experiences, while clearly informing current functioning and internal object-relations, are not the major focus of DIT. They may be included in the formulation shared with the patient so as to meaningfully frame his current difficulties in the context of his lived experience over time, but they are not a central component of the therapeutic process. Rather, given the brief nature of the therapy, the focus is on a core segment of the patient's interpersonal functioning that is closely connected with the presenting symptom(s).

The IPAF guides the therapist's interventions during the middle phase and provides the focus for helping the patient to begin to make some changes. It is through small changes in one circumscribed interpersonal area that shifts in functioning can often occur and that symptoms are alleviated. These developments rely on the therapist's unwavering and empathic attention to the IPAF. In practice this means that the therapist will actively redirect the patient back to the focus if the patient digresses from it and will actively work to understand with the patient why he might need to avoid the IPAF. Occasionally, the therapist will find that more than one interpersonal pattern needs to be addressed. Where this is the case, the therapist would discuss and agree this with the patient. When deciding what to focus on, it is important to bear in mind that DIT is a brief therapy that is not aiming to facilitate characterological change. Rather, the IPAF is selected in terms of its most immediate relevance to the onset of the patient's depression and/or anxiety.

Here-and-now focus

The "here-and-now" focus is central to DIT and denotes three related activities, namely the focus on *current affect*, on the patient's *current difficulties*, and on his *current relationship with the therapist*. We will now look at each of these in more detail.

Focus on affect

Throughout the therapy careful attention is devoted to the patient's affective state during the session, not least his pattern of affect regulation. The cognitive–affective structures of self and other representations regulate the patient's interpersonal exchanges, especially with significant attachment figures in the present. Helping the patient to become cognisant of what he feels, of the interpersonal triggers for particular feelings, and of how he manages these, is a core feature of DIT.

As this affective exploration takes place, the emotional state of the therapist is important to the patient's own emotional state. This is not on account of passive processes such as mirroring. Rather, it results from the patient's active use of the therapist's emotional expression in forming his appreciation of an event and using it to guide behavior. For example, a patient who was in thrall to a harsh superego, and who became very caught up in his mind with self-destructive accusations, responded with significant relief when a "confession" about a sexual transgression was normalized and responded to by the therapist with empathy and curiosity rather than admonishment. The function performed by the therapist here is that of transforming the patient's experience into something emotionally digestible. As she responds, the therapist thus provides the patient with an experience of being understood that enables him to gradually build up a sense that his own behavior is meaningful and communicative. The quality of these exchanges can contribute to laying the foundations for the patient's capacity to recognize and regulate affects, which will be less well developed in some patients.

The capacity to reflect on what we are feeling underscores our capacity to regulate affect (Fonagy et al., 2004). Each patient's pattern of affective arousal is different. Our understanding of this rests on a careful tracking of the patient's emotional state during the session. This tracking involves a number of related interventions as follows:

- *Help the patient to recognize his feelings as his own*: many patients come into therapy without any real sense of what they really feel. Helping them to label their feelings is often an essential first step in the process. This requires a shift away from the "why" of experience (often of concern to psychodynamic therapists) to the "what" of experience.

- *Help the patient to differentiate feelings from actions*: some patients, particularly those who struggle to represent their experience in their minds, can all too readily experience feelings as actions. The failure of the capacity to symbolize, to interpose thought between feeling and action, may render some feelings terrifying.

- *Facilitate discussion of the connection between feelings and actions*, which in turn facilitates self-understanding and awareness of motivations attributed to others (e.g. when I feel anxious I want to avoid being with you . . . I missed last week's session because I think you find me boring).

Focus on exploration of current difficulties

DIT focuses on the exploration of current difficulties in the patient's life rather than on trying to establish links to the childhood origins of these difficulties. Although some reconstructive interpretations are made during the course of DIT these are not considered to be a primary vehicle for facilitating change. Rather, the emphasis is placed on interventions that help the patient to feel he is working on difficulties that are live and current (in his current relationships, including that with the therapist) and over which he can effect a degree of change. The aim is thus to review the patient's experience related to the IPAF as much in the current as possible, that is, what the patient feels and is struggling with right now.

Focus on the therapeutic relationship

An important current relationship that is focused on in DIT is that with the therapist. DIT makes active use of the patient–therapist relationship to help the patient to explore the IPAF in the immediacy of this relationship (see Chapter 8). The relative balance placed in DIT between transference interpretations and other kinds of interventions is primarily dictated by the patient, moment-by-moment, since this kind of interpretation is a "high-risk, high-gain phenomenon" (Gunderson and Gabbard, 1999).

With some patients, for example those who have few current relationships, or those who struggle to report on relationships outside of therapy for defensive reasons, the transference relationship becomes a primary entry point into the patient's affective experience and his imaginative life (that is, his fantasies). For others, however, the report of their current relationships outside of therapy will be affectively charged and provide sufficient immediacy for the therapist to be able to engage the patient in a live exploration of the IPAF without needing to systematically elaborate these patterns at the level of the transference. The interpretation of the transference is thus guided by the extent to which the exploration of the IPAF is rendered more emotionally "persuasive" by this focus as opposed to a focus on what is happening on relationships outside of the therapy.

Focus on the patient's mind

A distinguishing feature of DIT is that it approaches the exploration of problematic interpersonal patterns not by addressing the patient's behavior, but through its consistent focus on the patient's conscious and unconscious mental states (beliefs, feelings, wishes, and thoughts) in himself and what he imagines or believes with conviction to be going on in the minds of others. The capacity to mentalize supports, in each of us, the daily struggle with what it means to have a mind. In some patients this capacity is severely undermined and this deficit may be regarded as central to their psychopathology, as in the case of borderline patients, for example (Bateman and Fonagy, 2006). In depressed and anxious patients, even if this deficit could not be described as characteristically central to their psychopathology in quite the same way, it is nevertheless the case that these patients do evidence failures of mentalization that contribute to their difficulties in relationships.

A central aim in DIT is to provide the patient with an experience of being with another person who is interested in thinking with him about what distresses him so as to stimulate the patient's own capacity for reflecting on his own experience. The goal is thus not only to work on an unconscious conflict, but also to use the focus on the IPAF to stimulate the patient's own capacity for thinking and feeling his experience.

This focus on the patient's state of mind is fundamental to DIT and it informs technique in so far as the helpfulness of the therapist's interventions (e.g. the interpretation of transference) is evaluated against the criterion of whether they help to stimulate the patient's capacity to represent his own subjective experience in relation to that of others, in the context of a problematic interpersonal relationship.

The DIT therapist is particularly interested in making explicit what has effectively become procedural so that the patient is then better able to effect change in how he manages his relationships. Working through the IPAF therefore involves not only challenging unthinking patterns of relating in attachment situations, through the central example of the IPAF, but also enhancing the patient's awareness of how his behavior and his affective state is driven by conscious and unconscious mental states. That is, the patient's social interactions and expressions of feeling will crucially depend on how he understands his own and others' motivation.

The IPAF is a particular locus of fixed interpretation. So, for example, say that there is in the patient's mind an unconscious expectation that "I am an unlovable person condemned to loneliness, the person

I want to be with is contemptuous of me, I will always be ashamed and humiliated; I need to protect myself by keeping a distance and pretending not to want a relationship." This will loosen its grip as mentalization increases through trying out different perspectives on the "evidence" in current, "hot" examples, especially through looking at sensitivities in relation to the therapist.

Therapeutic stance

The so-called analytic attitude is a core distinguishing feature of a psychodynamic approach. To a large extent—and we will qualify this shortly—this is also true of DIT.

Nowadays there is no consensually held notion of shared psychodynamic technique (Gabbard and Westen, 2003), such that even definitions of the analytic attitude are subject to variation across different schools of psychoanalysis. There is nevertheless a degree of consensus about the importance of the therapist being as unobtrusive as possible and of retaining a more neutral, relatively anonymous stance towards the patient that prioritizes reflection and interpretation over action. Such an attitude, of course, is in itself an intervention because patients will react differently, for example, to the therapist's interest in the meaning behind the patient's request for advice rather than its provision. The patient's reactions to the therapist then become the focus of exploration and provide opportunities for understanding the transference and, through this, the patient's internal world of relationships.

Keeping to an interpretative mode conveys to the patient, even if painfully, that difficult states of mind can be reflected upon with another person. This way of working has contributed to a caricature of the psychodynamic therapist as aloof and unemotional. This caricature is common, and while it may be true of some individual therapists, it is by no means true of the majority, and it would be incongruent with the more supportive, collaborative stance adopted by the DIT therapist. The therapist's aloofness is, in our view, unhelpful. Striving for "neutrality" and relative anonymity are important but should not result in emotional detachment. Rather than being aloof, the therapist should be actively engaged and emotionally attuned to the patient's subjective experience: she is also a participant in the therapeutic process and will experience strong feelings in response to the patient's communications.

The analytic attitude at its best—and as we define in DIT—is about a particular way of listening (see Chapter 7): the therapist empathizes with the patient's subjective experience while at the same time being curious about its unconscious meaning, rather than trying to solve problems or give advice. She also needs to be able to stand back from the interaction with the patient so as to reflect and comment on it, thereby helping the patient gain understanding of how he relates to others and thereby also modeling a reflective stance. Like all psychodynamic work this requires the therapist's ability to alternate between the temporary and partial identification of empathy and the return to the position of an observer to the interaction. It also requires a well-developed capacity for self-monitoring and self-scrutiny in order to reflect on and modify her responses in the moment and to note her own contribution to therapeutic impasses or enactments (see Chapter 8).

The DIT therapist thus adopts an involved, empathic, "supportively frustrating" manner. In other words, the core principles of an analytic attitude are adhered to but, where appropriate, an effort is made to contextualize the therapist's interventions. For example, if the patient reacts to the therapist's silence by feeling that the therapist is sitting in judgment of him, the therapist would convey acknowledgment and concern about the patient's experience of her silence, and might even explain that the silence is an attempt to allow the patient to say what is on his mind (a supportive intervention). The therapist would simultaneously remain focused on engaging the patient in identifying and exploring the state of mind triggered by her silence (an exploratory intervention that may be experienced as "frustrating" of the patient's wish to simply be rescued from what the silence exposes him to in his mind).

The therapist strives to adopt a "not-knowing" but curious stance that prioritizes the joint exploration of the patient's mental states as they relate to the identified interpersonal process that has been agreed as the focus of the therapy. Interpretations of deep unconscious material are generally avoided in favor of the facilitation and support of the patient's own capacity to stand back from his own immediate experience in order to be able to reflect on it.

From the outset the emphasis is on working collaboratively with the patient, especially in arriving at a formulation that provides a meaningful focus for the therapy. The therapist is explicit about the nature of DIT (she might, for example, also suggest to the patient that he reads the DIT user information leaflet—see Appendix 2), and of her understanding of the patient's problems, openly discussing and checking out the formulation with the patient, and jointly elaborating it in their formulation statement (see Chapter 5). The aim is to create the opportunity for the patient to participate actively in agreeing and understanding a focus for the work.

The patient's conscious as well as unconscious feedback on the therapy is important. This is provided through different "modes": concretely and directly through outcome monitoring forms, through conscious feedback, and indirectly through the narratives the patient brings that provide vehicles for unconscious communication about the therapy and the therapist.

It is important for the therapist to be receptive and responsive to both the patient's conscious and unconscious feedback and of the relationship between the two. If the patient questions the therapist's understanding, or her perception of the treatment, the therapist responds non-defensively, providing a clear, unambiguous account of how she has arrived at her understanding. The aim is to be as transparent as possible whilst being attuned to, and working with, the patient's need, where it arises, to control the therapist through projective processes.

Although the basic stance in DIT is thus an analytic one, rooted in an interest in the patient's conscious and unconscious communications, and in making use of the transference, the brevity of the treatment requires more activity on the part of the therapist. This might sometimes include, for example, "normalizing" experience by hypothetically disclosing what other people's thoughts and feelings might be in similar situations or through acknowledging the patient's progress and communicating hopefulness about progress. The therapist's self-disclosure is, however, generally discouraged.

Chapter 4

The Initial Phase

In any brief intervention the initial sessions are critical to the final outcome: the therapist not only has the task of engaging the patient so that he stays the course, but also needs to do so relatively rapidly given the brevity of the therapy. In large part engagement is facilitated through formulating a focus for the work that is both meaningful enough to the patient to engage him and that can be realistically addressed within the time limit.

The first four sessions in DIT are therefore devoted to identifying a focus for intervention that engages the patient to work actively on an area of his interpersonal functioning (the IPAF) in order to alleviate his more acute symptoms. In the next chapter we will focus in detail on how to formulate the IPAF. In this chapter we will review the aims and strategies of the *initial phase*, that is, sessions 1–4.

Engagement

In the initial phase one of the therapist's priorities is to actively work to engage the patient by developing a good therapeutic alliance. It can be all too easy to forget that initial sessions can be potentially "traumatic" for many patients, as Klauber (1981) rightly observed, as they take stock of painful aspects of themselves and of their current predicament, sometimes for the first time. This is all the more so when the focus of the therapist's exploration is on the patient's relationships and on his states of mind. This focus is invariably felt by the patient (even if only unconsciously) to implicitly direct attention to his contribution or responsibility for his current predicament. By contrast, labeling the patient's difficulties as an "illness" (for example, as the IPT therapist does) is often experienced as a relief for the patient who is then helped to depersonalize the problem (i.e., "It's not my fault").

If we accept that an assessment is inherently "traumatic" in this sense then it becomes incumbent on the therapist to create the conditions within which this trauma can be borne without the patient needing to take flight. This involves offering a measure of support and "orientation," as advocated by Sullivan (see Chapter 1), in order to foster "interpersonal security."

In order to minimize the likelihood of the patient's anxiety undermining the rapid development of the therapeutic alliance (which is crucial in a brief intervention), the DIT therapist provides some orientation to the patient by welcoming him, and introducing the aims of the initial sessions. The therapist will also ask questions more frequently than might be the case in more standard psychodynamic assessments. Although this stance is therefore more explicitly supportive, and hence structuring, the fundamental aim is one shared with all psychodynamic approaches: to help the patient gradually shift from a position where he is seeking help and relief from his symptoms to one where he is interested in meaning, in what is going on in his mind and in his relationships.

At this early stage it is important to assess whether the patient may require a strengthening of the supportive aspects of the therapeutic relationship in an explicit manner so as to engage him. The patient's responses to the therapist's interventions, to the silences and to the more emergent quality of the sessions are all informative. Assessing the patient's situation in relation to the feasibility of participating in a short-term treatment is important, as is ensuring that there are no significant implicit threats to the treatment being offered (see Chapter 2).

The therapist uses her experience of the patient's response to her in the session in order to identify what adaptations may be necessary to meet the needs of a patient who may have difficulty engaging with therapy. For example, some patients may have had little, if any, experience of another person helping them to make sense of what they feel. With such patients, to begin with, the work is often not about uncovering meaning; rather, it is about helping the patient to build a relationship within which he can articulate what he feels before he can begin to explore *why* he feels in a particular way.

The provision of more or less structure in the session will therefore be informed by the live experience with a particular patient, at a given point in time, and reviewed in every session.

Engaging the patient involves communicating respect for, and acceptance of, him. The therapist responds to the patient's presenting problems in a concerned, non-judgmental manner. This will be conveyed through the more prosodic features of speech such as tone of voice and also through:

- Asking clarifying questions so as to understand the patient's perspective without making assumptions: "You said the relationship with X was 'less of a burden.' What do you have in mind when you say that?"

- Communicating empathic understanding in response to the patient's conscious and unconscious communications: "When I just asked you about your mother your whole demeanor changed: you stiffened and you began to speak very fast as if you felt the pressure to answer me, and yet you also seemed to just want to move away from thinking about this with me."

- Respecting the patient's need for defenses: "Ensuring you insulate yourself from others is a way of protecting yourself from this feeling of rejection. Given what you have been through in your life I can see that you feel this is essential."

- Maintaining an engaged, active, and realistically optimistic attitude that conveys support for the patient's development and therapeutic goals: "As I listen to you talking about what you want for yourself I can sense your commitment to making some changes in your life. Even though we both know that this will be challenging, your motivation to do so comes across and is a real strength."

- Using collaborative language: "*We* will work on this focus together and one of my tasks will be to ensure that we keep to this focus."

- Validating the patient's experience as understandable given the circumstances: "It is understandable that you should feel so mistrustful and alert to danger since your assault—it was a deeply unsettling experience."

Listening out for "cautionary tales"

The initial sessions are critical to the course of DIT for the simple reason that without a patient in the room there is no therapy. An important way of fostering the therapeutic alliance is through containing the patient's anxiety about engaging in therapy and the threats this is felt to pose.

Communicating clearly at the outset the boundaries and frame of the therapy and its nature is necessary so as to give the patient a sense that he can understand what is being offered and can give meaningful consent to it. This is the basis for a collaborative relationship. However, for some patients the nature of their anxiety about starting therapy may not be contained sufficiently by clarifying these important parameters. Some patients will need more explicit indications from the therapist that she understands just how fearful they feel at the prospect of therapy, for example, through acknowledging the challenge that making change in the patient's life implies (e.g. "It's not easy to change and I can understand why you might not want to do it at all").

More importantly, however, the anxiety becomes manageable if the patient can be helped to reflect on the unconscious anxieties about the therapy and the therapist, and if the therapist is experienced and capable of tolerating the patient's feelings about this ("You have clearly conveyed to me that your experience of being helped has always been negative: you invariably trust another person, then feel exposed, and then somehow neglected. Even though you keep reassuring me—and yourself too—that talking to a therapist will be different, I could well understand if in fact you were feeling very concerned that this purportedly helpful relationship will deteriorate into this painful, familiar pattern").

A key task in the initial sessions is therefore to listen out for the patient's "cautionary tales" (Ogden, 1992), that is, his unconscious anxieties about developing a relationship with the therapist that will reflect particular expectations of himself and of other people. The anxieties are typically communicated through the interpersonal narratives (INs) that the patient brings. The quality of the fantasies the patient has about us is vitally important to the viability and outcome of DIT. At the outset many prospective patients are likely to turn to us with a mixture of fear and hope that activates latent fantasies regarding authority figures and caregivers, fantasies into which we will be uncon-sciously fitted. The patients most difficult to help in time-limited ther-apy are those with persecutory fantasies that shape virtually all aspects of their mind because they relate to the world with fantasies organized around controlling, tormenting, or rejecting the object before they then run the risk of becoming the victim of fantasized retaliatory attacks.

More typically the patient's anxieties will reflect the belief that rela-tionships will inevitably become painful, disappointing, unreliable, overly sexualized, etc. Many patients, but by no means all, arrive at the consultation in a state of need, looking for an authoritative person to relieve the distress. The underlying initial transference may therefore be to a powerful, omniscient parental figure. In turn, this may set up a conflict between the wish for, and fear of, a dependent relationship as it immediately establishes the therapeutic relationship as unequal in the patient's mind.

Being able to accurately identify these cautions and convey under-standing of them to the patient draws his attention in an immediate way to his anxieties. It also allows the therapist to give the patient an experience of the kind of reflection that will take place within the therapy whilst testing out the patient's capacity to make use of it (see also Chapter 2).

It is helpful and containing for the patient if the therapist is able to articulate these anxieties early on, so that they can then be incorpo-rated into the formulation of the IPAF—sometimes the representation of self and other that underpins the cautionary tale becomes the essence of the IPAF. In the following clinical vignettes we can see how for each patient an important dimension of their internal experience emerges through the narratives that are recounted and the therapist's understanding leads to the articulation of distinctive cautionary tales.

Case examples of "cautionary tales"

Mr F. arrived late and flustered for his first session. He complained about the traffic and was evidently angry with a driver whom he said had taken his place at a meter. He referred to the driver in derogatory terms. Although he was apologetic about his lateness, the therapist nevertheless immediately felt on guard as if she was somehow to blame.

Mr F. was one of five children. He spoke about a rather deprived early childhood where both parents had been unemployed and the family struggled to make ends meet. Mr F.'s depression coincided with a stressful work situation where he was "moved sideways." He felt bitter about this decision and had since lost all interest in his work. He thought that he had been discriminated against because he had not gone to a good university.

As the therapist listened she thought that his narrative about the difficulty with parking contained an important "caution," namely about the extent to which the patient was preoccupied with how much space the object would have in her mind for him. This alerted the therapist to the likelihood that he might experience her, in the transference, as favoring another in her mind who would be seen as taking up the space that should rightfully belong to him. Moreover, the therapist was also alerted to the underlying grievance and his difficulty in taking any responsibility for his part in this dynamic. This, in turn, helped the therapist to speak with the patient about this core anxiety as he approached the prospect of therapy.

Another patient, Ms Y., who was referred because she was seized by panic when she had to present her work in public, also arrived late for her first session. She was duly very apologetic and the therapist sensed her considerable unease in the session as Ms Y. could barely look at her. Early on in the session Ms Y. recounted an incident from her university days when she had agreed to present her work to her peer group, but when she arrived in the seminar she felt frozen and had stammered, which had only made her feel worse. She had then withdrawn to her room for weeks feeling as if she had "leprosy," as she put it.

Towards the end of the session, after picking up further confirmatory evidence, both from the stories the patient recounted and the therapist's own countertransference, the therapist returned to this story as a marker for how exposed the patient was feeling in the session. She said that one risk they both needed to keep in mind was that she might experience the therapy a bit like the seminar, and fear being similarly exposed and humiliated by the therapist. If that were the case then her only solution might be to withdraw from the therapy, a bit as she had perhaps done by arriving late and hence limiting her exposure to the therapist's evaluation of her.

What do we need to know in order to formulate a dynamic focus for intervention?

Before we turn to how to formulate we need first to establish the range of information that the therapist is interested in so as to arrive at a formulation that can then be shared with the patient.

History-taking versus history-making

Psychiatric and psychotherapy assessments are structured around eliciting a patient's history but this can be done in different ways. Psychiatrists typically question the patient systematically about his childhood history his sexual and relationship history, his occupational history, and his previous treatments. A great deal of information is thus collected. Asking about a patient's occupational history or knowing about his sexual history may yield valuable information that will inform an understanding of the problem. Nevertheless, reading through standard psychiatric reports and then meeting the patient in question it soon becomes apparent that this type of detailed, factual information about a patient tells us comparatively little about his capacity to use therapy or, indeed, about his problems and their dynamic meaning.

In order to gain a more in-depth perspective of the patient, we need to pay attention to the *process* of the assessment. In other words, we must be attuned to how the patient constructs his narrative (i.e., the form as opposed to the content of what the patient communicates) and what use he makes of us in doing so. Throughout the early stages of DIT it is therefore important for the therapist to reflect on what is happening between her and the patient and consider some of the following: how does the patient relate to the therapist? How does the patient describe his experiences? What feelings are triggered in the therapist during this process? The answers to such questions are as important as, and often far more informative than, the biographical information collected.

The relationship that evolves during these initial sessions between patient and therapist is important on practical and epistemological grounds. From a purely practical point of view no meaningful assessment or formulation of the patient's difficulties could be arrived at without attention and effort to establish a good working alliance with the patient. If the patient cannot trust the therapist, nor experience empathic concern on her part, he is unlikely to engage fully in the sessions or in the subsequent proposed therapy.

There are also theoretical reasons for the privileged space accorded here to the relationship between therapist and patient. Contemporary epistemologists argue that all knowledge is a process by which the knower actively organizes and shapes what is perceived and thought, and thereby constructs what is known. Knowledge of a patient then represents the outcome of a dynamic interaction between knower and known, between subject and object. The therapist needs to be mindful of the fact that the knowledge gathered in these early sessions is inevitably, in one sense, subjective.

What is being described here is not "history-taking" as such rather, the emphasis is on "history-making" (Hirschberg, 1993), that is, on the importance of addressing how the patient organizes and constructs his account of his difficulties as he engages with the therapist. It can indeed be helpful to comment on this explicitly during early sessions. For example, as well as commenting on any contradictions or omissions in a patient's account, the therapist might take note of how much or how little detail is offered, whether the narrative is difficult or easy to follow, or whether the patient appears preoccupied with particular relationships that cause his concerns to be related in a muddled or incoherent fashion.

The way the patient presents his history will give us important clues about his capacity to think about himself in relation to others and about others in relation to himself; that is, it tells us something about his capacity for self-reflection. When we listen to the way the patient constructs his narrative we are paying attention to how he presents his relationships with the significant figures in his life. For example, if there are difficulties in a relationship we note whether the patient shows evidence of an awareness that how he feels about the difficult situation may be different to how the other person feels about it.

Coherent narratives, which are associated with secure attachments, tend to include an acknowledgement of conflict, pain, and mixed feelings; in speaking about such difficulties the patient demonstrates an appreciation of the complexity of his own and other people's motivations. By contrast, those narratives typically associated with an insecure attachment status reveal more unnoticed contradiction, denial, confusion, or overwhelming negative affects such as anger or fear. The patient may, for example, recount abusive experiences and yet talk about them in a very cut-off manner, dismissing their significance, or he may relate a very confusing story, leaving us feeling that he is still in the thick of negative emotional experience and cannot recognize or have perspective on it.

Listening in this way is very different to "taking a history." The skill lies in managing to combine this very specialized type of listening (see Chapter 7), which is the hallmark of analytic listening, with a capacity to weave in and out of the patient's narrative and cover certain areas of the patient's life and functioning that we need to know about in order to meaningfully assess his capacity to make use of DIT. For example, the patient may well respond to an interpretation about his internal world and this may lead us to conclude that he could use DIT. However, if we know nothing or little about who is actually in his current life and who could support him through the demands of therapy, we may be arriving at a wrong conclusion. Some patients are unable to manage the space in-between the sessions if they have few or no support systems. It is therefore imperative that by the end of the initial phase we know something not only about the primitive figures that populate the patient's internal world, but also about who exists in the patient's external world and the quality of those relationships (see below).

In order to be in a position to formulate we need to gather relevant information in the following domains.

History of the presenting problem: the symptom/problem from the patient's point of view

To begin with we need to take a history of the problem and its time line (see Box 4.1). The aim is to create an understanding of the onset of the difficulties that bring the patient into therapy. For many patients the problem will have developed gradually, with a succession of events contributing to their recognition that there is a problem. Others may recognize that there is a problem that is getting worse, but be unclear how it started or why a preferable situation may have deteriorated. In such cases there may be stressful life events or major changes associated with the onset of the problem, as well as changes with its intensity. In many cases the problem, which is ostensibly the reason why the patient has been referred or has actively sought therapy, may not be, in fact, the source of distress. Rather, it acts as a distraction.

The question "why now?" is a most important one to clarify: it is useful to establish why a patient presents for help at this particular

Box 4.1 Assessment of the problem/symptoms

This will include:

- Its nature as perceived by the patient (e.g. is it experienced as "symptoms" that need managing or as a problem in relationships?)
- Its origins (when did it start?)
- Its course over time, bearing in mind modulating and exacerbating variables (what makes it better or worse?)
- Its interpersonal context (how do the patient's relationships affect the problem/symptoms and how are they affected by it?)
- Its severity (what are the risks to the patient and/or others?)

time, as this may give some indication as to what other difficulties may be occurring in his life. This exploration is important not only because it provides the therapist with information relevant to the eventual formulation, but also because the process of examining the course of one's difficulties over time can implicitly help the patient gain some perspective over his problem, and to an extent perhaps increase its predictability and so his sense of perceived control over his life.

The family history

The family history includes information about the constitution of the nuclear as well as extended family. Information about the extended family is often very important as it can lead to an exploration of how particular patterns or dynamics may be repeating themselves across generations. The family composition typically includes information about who is in the family, deaths (including miscarriages, terminations, and stillbirths), marriages, divorces, or separations.

Medical history and the patient's bodily self

If the patient presents with some physical problems which appear to be connected with depression and/or anxiety, taking a very brief medical history will be important to ascertain exactly what is happening in relation to the patient's experience of his physical self. However, such a history should not overshadow the more important exploration of the meaning attributed by the patient to any physical problems and how these affect his perception of himself or how they may be used interpersonally (e.g. to ensure proximity to an attachment figure: "If I'm ill then she will not leave me").

Our patients bring their minds *and* their bodies to psychotherapy, yet it is surprising how often we neglect the body both in ongoing therapy and at the assessment stage. A rich source of information about the patient's experience of himself can be discerned through carefully taking note of how he relates to his physicality because the actual or fantasized limits of the body influence how we relate to ourselves and to others. Visual or auditory impairment, for example, not only affects the individual on a pragmatic level, but also profoundly influences the confidence with which he approaches the world and, importantly, the way others relate to him.

We can begin to reflect on the patient's subjective experience of his body by observing his use of the physical space in the consulting room and the way he experiences himself in his body. For example, a very tall patient may walk into our room stooped while another may walk into the room and bump into the furniture. It is seldom appropriate at the assessment stage to comment on striking features of someone's physicality since at this early stage any thoughts we will have about the matter are likely to be highly speculative. Referring to them may also feel very intrusive to the patient. However, feeling free to note in our own mind these perceptions and reactions to the patient's physical presence may provide yet another source of information that can assist us in the task of formulating.

Mapping the interpersonal landscape

The patient's internal world of object relationships

An important task in these early sessions is to map out the patient's characteristic interpersonal style through closely exploring his experience of significant relationships past and present (see Figure 4.1). The therapist's basic stance during these early sessions is one of curiosity about the patient's subjective experience of his interpersonal world so as to tease out recurring relational and affective patterns that are typically structured around a "self" and "other" representation. The richest

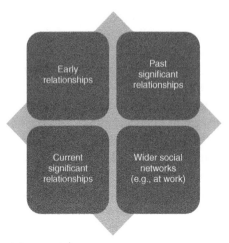

Figure 4.1 The interpersonal map.

source of information about the dominant qualities of these unconscious representations can be gleaned from the stories the patient
reports of his relationships, what we refer to here as "interpersonal
narratives" (INs).

From the outset, the emphasis in DIT is on trying to locate the problem in an interpersonal context, that is, to understand how the manifest problem (e.g. depression) can be approached as a manifestation of
a circumscribed, recurring interpersonal pattern. This requires
focused attention on helping the patient to report INs, which will
allow the therapist eventually to formulate the patient's internal world
of relationships as the basis for helping him to understand his subjective experience of relationships. Here, the focus is placed on *recurring
interpersonal scenarios* rather than on the actual protagonists involved
and the specifics of the situation.

In order to assess the quality of the patient's relationships, the therapist thus encourages the patient to not only talk about the problem as
seen by the patient, but also provide narratives about his relationships,
past and present. For example, if the patient is focusing narrowly on a
description of symptoms, the therapist sensitively acknowledges their
distressing nature, but also enquires about the interpersonal context in
which the symptoms occur or fluctuate.

As the patient tells us his story we begin to listen out for patterns in his relationships that will assist us in building a schematic picture of his internal world. It is helpful to note what repetitive conflicts emerge as we explore these relationships, for example, whether the patient repeatedly engages in relationships where he is submissive or where he feels secretly triumphant over other people. Likewise, we note which dynamics are absent, for example, whether relationships are reported to always be conflict-free. Omissions and emphases are often telling. Some patients display from the outset reluctance to talk about a particular period of their lives. For example, the patient's narrative may be skewed in favor of detailed accounts of his childhood experiences, or the patient may only talk about his present life and gloss over past history. Omissions or cursory descriptions should always alert us to the operation of resistance. In these situations the patient may be helped to explore a difficult period in his life if we can recognize first that he feels in some danger if he reveals or thinks, say, things about his early childhood.

There are two key questions that we need to be able to tentatively answer by the end of the first four sessions:

- What kind of relationship(s) does the patient typically create?
- How does this relate to the presenting symptoms?

We are therefore interested in formulating the relationship models that organize the patient's experience, modulate affect and direct behavior, and that are meaningfully connected with the onset and maintenance of symptoms. Recurring interpersonal configurations alert us to internalized object relationships that have taken root in the patient's internal world. The patient's pattern of relating can become entrenched such that he can only function by adopting a very specific role in relation to the other, or he filters what he perceives in highly predictable ways, for example, the patient who always hears criticism even when praised or sets up the other as invariably neglectful.

In asking the patient questions about a range of relationships (see Figure 4.2) one of our aims is to gain some sense of who the patient identifies with, both consciously and unconsciously, focusing on building a preliminary sketch of those qualities that have been assimilated or repudiated. A helpful question in this respect is to ask the patient what

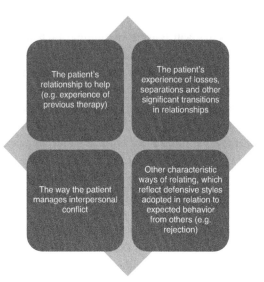

Figure 4.2 Interpersonal contexts yielding information about key attachment patterns.

his father and mother were/are like respectively. If the patient gives a very global reply, for example, "They were good parents," we can prompt him to be more specific, perhaps even to think of a few adjectives that best describe the parents. This exploration not only begins to put some flesh on the bones of the various significant figures in the patient's life, but the quality of the patient's descriptions is also informative because it gives some clues as to whether we are dealing with a predominantly borderline or neurotic personality organization.[1]

Patients with a more borderline characterological structure tend to portray others in global, dichotomous terms reflecting a split between their overall goodness or badness. Alternatively, they portray significant others in terms of the function they serve in the patient's life, that is, more as part-objects, devoid of their own autonomy and omnipotently controlled by the patient. Neurotic patients, on the other hand, tend to provide more balanced, multidimensional accounts of other

---

[1] DIT has not been developed for the treatment of BPD, but it is by no means uncommon to see patients who are referred because they are depressed and/or anxious who also present with borderline features.

people, revealing some appreciation of their distinct qualities, separate from the self, even if their view of the other may also be distorted by defensive processes such as projection.

In these early sessions we are therefore simultaneously thinking about the quality of the object relationships and making inferences about the level of maturity of these relationships, that is, whether the patient relates to whole- or part-objects and the patient's capacity to be separate from others. In this respect, it is important to make a distinction between a "narcissistic involvement" where the other is an appendage or extension of the self and a mature "object relationship" where the other is seen as separate from the self (Mason, 2000). It is helpful to consider too whether the self is experienced as cohesive or vulnerable to fragmentation if others are not available.

As we listen we are looking for evidence of the patient's ability to confide, to trust, and to see others as potentially helpful, as opposed to feeling paranoid and mistrustful of others' intentions towards the self. Having friends is encouraging, but it does not guarantee a capacity to genuinely engage with others as separate from the self. For example, the patient may relate internally to their so-called friends as no more than "cloned confirmations of the self" (Bolognini, 2006)—that is, narcissistic satellites that hold the self together but do not allow for the other's separate existence.

Keeping in mind the external reality of the patient's interpersonal context

DIT's emphasis on the importance of our actual attachments to mental well-being orients the therapist to the importance of the patient's *current*, external context. This will include the world of social networks, work, and/or education. It also includes attention to the impact of race, culture, disability, sexuality, and unemployment on people's experience of themselves with others.

In addition to eliciting a relationship history, which will enable us to build a picture of the patient's internal world, it is therefore important to also assess the patient's wider social networks (including their educational and/or employment interpersonal contexts) and the quality and patterning of the interactions between the patient and their friends/acquaintances (e.g. issues of relationship to authority, dependency and autonomy, trust, etc.). This provides yet another source of information to assist us in identifying recurring interpersonal configurations, and hence a possible focus for the work.

The patient's external relationships and the availability of support, or otherwise, for the patient's wish to engage in therapy also deserves consideration. With more psychically fragile patients the question of who will support them during therapy needs to be carefully considered. Lack of support from work or family may undermine further a fragile therapeutic alliance and tenuous motivation for change. For the most disturbed patients with a proneness to acting out, special provision may need to be made to ensure they have additional professional supports for the duration of DIT.

Using the attachment styles questionnaire

In the first session, or the following one (depending on the degree of distress and detail in the immediate presentation), the exploration of the patient's characteristic stance towards relationships is opened up and facilitated by suggesting that he reads and chooses one of the attachment style statements below (Hazan and Shaver, 1987, supplemented by Bartholomew and Horowitz, 1991). This can be done along with the other questionnaires that the patient will be asked to fill in as part of outcome monitoring.

The patient is asked to rate each statement, on the scales, so that this can begin a discussion with the therapist about his usual behavior in, and feelings about, close relationships. These ratings are then revisited in the *ending phase*. Their review provides an opportunity for reflecting on the change that has occurred (which may well be outside awareness, as pervasive attachment assumptions or attitudes are usually more implicit than conscious), and any further changes that the patient would like to work towards in the future. For the most part the scores on these attachment descriptors, unsurprisingly, show little change over the course of sixteen sessions, but what can, and often does, change is the patient's appraisal of their characteristic patterns (i.e., less distorted by defenses) and of how he would like to change.

The statements are:

A. It is easy for me to become emotionally close to others. I am comfortable depending on them and having them depend on me.

I don't worry about being alone or having others not accept me. [This corresponds to a "secure" tendency in relation to adult attachment, where the person is relatively positive about both self and other.]

B. I am uncomfortable getting close to others. I want emotionally close relationships, but I find it difficult to trust others completely, or to depend on them. I worry that I will be hurt if I allow myself to become too close to others. [This corresponds to a "fearful" stance, where the person is relatively negative about both self and other and, while feeling vulnerable, feels unsafe in a dependent relationship.]

C. I want to be completely emotionally intimate with others, but I often find that others are reluctant to get as close as I would like. I am uncomfortable being without close relationships, but I sometimes worry that others don't value me as much as I value them. [This characterizes a "preoccupied" attachment style, the patient being negative about self and ostensibly positive about the other; it would be expected to be associated with intense but anxious relationships, which may also be ambivalent and unstable.]

D. I am comfortable without close emotional relationships. It is very important to me to feel independent and self-sufficient, and I prefer not to depend on others or have others depend on me. [This captures a "dismissing" attachment style, the patient being positive about the self and negative about the other; it suggests distance and an unconsciously defensive stance of self-sufficiency. It may be associated with actual denigration of others and relationships, or apparent lack of interest in them.]

The patient is asked to rate how like him each statement is, giving a profile across the four prototypical stances which delineates his predominant approach to relationships and closeness.

◆ Relationship maps dominated by Style A are characterized by being balanced (selective, flexible), reversible, stable (consistent over time and progressive, developing positively over time).

The other patterns are typically inflexible in structure within a relationship, and repetitive across different contexts.

Table 4.1 Attachment style rating scale

	Not at all like me			Somewhat like me			Very much like me
Style A	1	2	3	4	5	6	7
Style B	1	2	3	4	5	6	7
Style C	1	2	3	4	5	6	7
Style D	1	2	3	4	5	6	7

- Style B relationships are characterized by perceived dangers and risks, the patient is fearful of intimacy and can be quite socially avoidant, or volatile as the conflict between getting close and having to escape gets repetitively played out.

- Style C is characterized by a preoccupation with relationships, bringing others too close to the self and generating unstable and self-focused structures where the patient imagines knowing more about the feelings of others than is justified by circumstances. This can be seen as an effort to feel more in control of and less confused by intense involvements with "over-thinking" in the absence of a real understanding of the feelings and motivations of self or other, despite a continual need to engage.

- Style D relationships are distancing and often quite stable but inflexible. There may be considerable selfishness and thoughtlessness, where others are rarely seen clearly as "three-dimensional" real figures and there is little conscious emotional investment.

The therapist should be particularly wary of problematic combinations of styles. For example, a style that combines preoccupation with relationships and fearfulness of them often characterizes individuals who are exceptionally vulnerable to rejection. Other unhelpful "combined" styles include that of distancing with preoccupation, where the strategies dictated by these styles contradict one another. More positive are combinations of Style A with other styles. An endorsement of Style A and denial of affinity to the other styles is likely to reflect a pattern of denial.

The patient's cultural context

We do not develop in isolation. From the moment of birth we are a part of a family system but also of wider systems, such as the culture we are born into. This wider system needs to be integrated into our understanding of the patient's presenting problem and of his relationships.

The internal world is always in a dynamic interaction with the external world. Although there is never a direct correspondence between external and internal, as what is internal reflects the operation of defensive processes that distort what is taken in from the outside, our assessments and formulations need to reflect the reality of our patients' lives as much as what they idiosyncratically make of this reality. In order to have the best possible understanding of our patients and of their needs we need to be curious about the world they live in externally. If we do not ask about it, we may never know, and we can jump to erroneous conclusions.

Culture is especially important because the very notions of self, of separation, and of individuation that are so commonplace within Western models of therapy may not be as relevant for other cultures. In the West the individuated self is the goal of therapy. It is a self that values differentiation. In the East the relational self is more permeable and we encounter more fluid self–other boundaries; the unit of identity is not an internal representation of the other but of the family or community.

The relationship with the therapist will also be influenced by cultural factors. By virtue of our own cultural identifications or our race we may find it easier to relate to some patients than others, and the same will apply to our patients. Being open and receptive to these transferences and countertransferences is essential to a good assessment. Patients do not always seek likeness in their therapists with respect to cultural background. Instead some actively seek difference and in so doing may be communicating something very important about their own cultural identifications. For example, one mixed race young woman specifically requested a white therapist. In the therapy it soon became clear that the "white" self was good and the "black" self was bad, hence she defensively wanted to identify herself with the white therapist.

How many relationships need to be explored before sharing a formulation with the patient?

As a general rule, all significant attachments past and present deserve exploration. It is best to start with an exploration of the patient's significant current relationships and work backwards to the patient's early experiences. For each relationship, the therapist engages the patient in thinking about the perceived quality of these relationships and how they impact on the patient's experience of himself.

It is important to elicit at least one detailed account of some important current interpersonal interactions in which "the attachment system" has been activated, for example, an argument with a partner. In this context the therapist can focus on identifying common communication difficulties, explore any open conflict with intense affect and understand its outcomes, identify and point to ambiguous, indirect nonverbal communication, point to dramatically distorted assumptions (i.e., that one has communicated or that one has understood), highlight problematic communication patterns (e.g. silent closing off communication and repetitive statements—"I know that I am no good"), and point to risky communication by listening for the assumptions that the patient makes about others' thoughts or feelings, including the therapist's.

Identifying aims and negotiating the therapeutic content

All the information that is gleaned from exploring the various dimensions of the patient's experience, as outlined above, contributes to the formulation of the IPAF. In the next chapter we focus exclusively on how this is done in DIT. For now we want to continue sketching out the overall trajectory for the initial phase, where, once the focus is agreed with the patient, an important task during session 4 is to engage the patient in articulating the aims for the therapy. This may well not be familiar territory for some psychodynamic clinicians, but the identification of meaningful and realistic goals is important in a time-limited intervention. It creates a helpful opportunity for the therapist to engage the patient at the outset in working towards change and promotes hopefulness.

The process of identifying goals begins with the therapist enquiring explicitly about what the patient hopes to achieve. Many patients will give very diffuse, general answers to this question such as "I want to be happy." The challenge is to help the patient to translate this general wish into something more specific and interpersonal such as "I want to be able to communicate to others what I need from them"—a capacity that would contribute to their sense of happiness.

When discussing aims the patient's resources need to be considered along with his vulnerabilities so as to help the patient to reflect on his expectations of therapy and introduce some realism about what might and might not be achievable. It is also timely to acknowledge here the patient's strengths.

With some patients the most realistic goal is to set in motion a process of understanding or of "working towards" some change in relationships rather than achieving an observable change in their relationships over the sixteen sessions.

For others a stated goal(s) may well conflict with an unstated one(s). Where this is the case, the therapist therefore also needs to communicate understanding that, in addition to the stated aims, there might be less conscious aims that oppose change. For example, a patient might ostensibly say that he would like to gain better understanding of why his marriage is failing, but the unconscious aim is to recruit the therapist into supporting his position against the partner.

How much information does the patient need about DIT in order to consent to it?

Therapy is not the place for a seminar on how therapy works, but neither is it unreasonable for patients to want to find out what we think about their difficulties and how we think we can help them. During the initial sessions some patients will ask about the therapy and how it works. Such a question may, of course, also mask anxiety about engaging in the process and this needs to be explored, but we have a duty to inform our patients of the service they are receiving, just like any other service. Patients both have a right to know and are possibly anxious for their own individual reasons.

Some patients may well be preoccupied with whether they are "mad" or "bad," or whether we think they will get better or not. It is important to avoid colluding with the patient's wish for a definitive answer to his problem by offering detailed replies on this front, which in any event could only be partial and tentative at such an early stage. Nevertheless, it is part of the therapist's responsibility to convey to the patient an understanding of his predicament and how the proposed therapy might help him with this. Only interpreting his questions as reflecting anxiety about the process, or his fear that he might be going mad or is "bad," is unhelpful, though such speculations will be true for some patients. In our responses we can both acknowledge the actual question and give some opinion as well as attend to the anxiety that may reside behind the question.

In DIT the therapist is direct and transparent about her understanding of the patient's difficulties and how the therapy will help him. At the end of session 4, or earlier where indicated, the therapist will provide the patient with sufficient direct information about the therapy (including its risks and benefits) so as to make consent meaningful (see Appendix 2 for a sample information leaflet about DIT).

It is helpful to personalize the explanation of the treatment rationale by linking it to the patient's own history and current experiences. This minimizes the risk of becoming unhelpfully intellectual and increases the likelihood of engaging the patient in the treatment process. It is also helpful to manage expectations by stressing the difficulties involved in changing long-established patterns and pointing to the challenge that the patient is about to undertake.

In session 4 the therapist will also agree a verbal contract with the patient, which will include specification of the following:

1. The affective–interpersonal context of the intervention.

2. The short-term duration (16 sessions once a week for about 50 minutes).

3. The problem area that will be targeted.

4. The crisis management plan where appropriate.

5. The agreement for session-by-session outcome monitoring.

Some patients passively accept what is offered. In such instances the therapist encourages the patient to reflect on his reactions to the proposed therapy and its general focus on feelings and relationships to enlist his more active participation in the process.

As we mentioned earlier, it is not necessary to enter into lengthy explanations about how DIT purports to help the patient, but it is essential to provide some brief guidance on the differential expectations of both therapist and patient so as to orient the patient to the particular style of therapy in sessions to come. The therapist might say something along these lines:

> Now that we have agreed a focus for our work I want to tell you about how we will work together. Each week I will leave it up to you to talk about the things that are on your mind. We have already identified a specific area in your relationships where there is room for change and I will try to keep us

focused on this because we will only be meeting for another 12 sessions. I am interested not only in what happens in your relationships between sessions, but also in your feelings about these events. This includes feelings about me, our relationship, or the therapy. It may feel difficult to raise this with me, but it will be important for us to think together about what may be on your mind in this respect.

Managing risk and self-harm

The management of risk in DIT is no different to what all therapists do when faced with a patient who is at risk of harming himself and/or others: the priority is to ensure safety. If the patient presents with a risk of self-harm, it is important to engage him at this early stage in jointly identifying how he will access help when in a crisis and putting into place additional supports, as necessary. The risk of self-harm is not constant and may itself fluctuate over the course of the therapy such that this requires a continuous, session-by-session assessment of the patient's state of mind. With more disturbed patients it is vital to carry out an assessment of risk during breaks in the treatment and to make arrangements for additional support when required.

Having stressed the importance of ensuring the patient's safety, it is also the case that in the area of mental health we inhabit a risk-averse culture where the need to act so as to pre-empt the patient's acting out can sometimes unhelpfully preclude reflection on the conscious and unconscious *meaning* of the patient's suicidal thoughts or violent fantasies (i.e., their interpersonal function) (see Briggs et al., 2008). It is therefore essential to consider not only how to keep the patient safe, but also what might be giving rise to an increase in risk: is the therapist pushing the patient too much? Is the patient trying in some way to attack the therapist? Is the self-harm a response to a separation? As well as complying with the service's governance structures for the management of risk, the DIT therapist should therefore not abandon her capacity to reflect on the unconscious meaning of the risky behavior and try to engage the patient in reflecting on it.

Managing the frame and the setting

The therapist strives to establish and maintain a consistent therapeutic frame, setting out clearly, at the outset, the parameters within which the treatment will take place (setting; frequency and length of sessions; limits of confidentiality; expectations of the patient; arrangements/ cover over breaks). Sometimes there will be pressures from the patient to change the frame. It is important to evaluate the meaning of the patient's requests for modifications to the parameters of the therapy as the basis for responding to such requests.

The therapist endeavors to be receptive to the patient's conscious and unconscious experience of the setting and its boundaries, and to help him to articulate this experience. This is so as to ensure that the agreement to the therapy and its boundaries is rooted in an explora-tion of the patient's conscious and unconscious feelings and fantasies about the therapy.

When managing forms of acting out in relation to the setting (by the patient, therapist, or both), the therapist strives to maintain (or regain) a reflective stance, but may also need to set clear limits where necessary (e.g. if the patient's behavior undermines the viability of the treatment).

Managing the frame involves the management of interruptions in the therapy by preparing the patient for planned interruptions (e.g. holiday breaks) and, once again, helping him to explore his conscious and unconscious responses to both planned and unplanned breaks. This exploration needs to be linked to the IPAF, where relevant, and is not carried out for its own sake.

The use of outcome monitoring and video/ audiotaping of sessions

In developing DIT we have been pragmatic in a number of ways, one of which is to embed the protocol in the discipline of routinely measur-ing outcomes. This is by no means standard practice within psycho-dynamic approaches. Like manuals and competences, we can now also add outcome monitoring to our list of "non-analytic-self" antigens, which are experienced as intruders and are repudiated by the "psychic immune system" (Britton, 2003). At its best, this kind of monitoring is construed as an intrusion into the therapeutic process or it is felt to be irrelevant because the measures used are often (and with good reason) considered inappropriate to the change process that dynamic app-roaches are trying to support. At worst the antipathy results from a strongly held belief in the effectiveness of the treatment being offered (Busch et al., 2009), which does not need to be evidenced beyond the clinical observation of the clinician and other like-minded colleagues. But as Busch and Milrod observe:

> Clinical lore and observation can be highly biased, as the subjectivity of the observer can override an accurate assessment of a patient's improvement. . . . Psychoanalysts pride themselves on their awareness of the impact of fantasy and wishful thinking during their treatments, but minimize the impact of such factors on their subjective assessment of their own clinical outcomes. Identification with powerful and respected leaders and theoreticians in the field can colour a more objective assessment of treatment effectiveness. In our wish to be therapeutic and our belief in our treatment, it is all too easy to disregard patients who were treatment failures. (Busch and Milrod, 2010: 310)

The aversion to outcome monitoring is also fuelled by our narcissism: outcome monitoring can understandably feel like a kind of personal monitoring and a deterioration in the patient's scores can feel like a crushing judgment of our competence (Okiishi et al., 2003). But to insist that only the therapist treating the patient can evaluate the results of psychodynamic treatment is to propose a closed loop system. Sophistication is necessary to evaluate patient reports in the consulting room as well as part of conducting outcome research. However, if sophistication becomes a euphemism for a policy that insists outcome can only be accurately judged by those committed to a particular form of treatment, confidence by the service users, the general public, and the scientific community will be eroded.

We take the view that despite the limitations of questionnaires in detecting meaningful and sometimes subtle changes, it is nevertheless good practice to monitor treatment outcomes, just as it is to tape sessions and have a supervisor listen to them. This kind of "monitoring" could be more helpfully construed as additional feedback for the therapist and, as such, another form of support to the therapist to help her to reflect on the course of therapy. Our experience on the ground has been that after some initial anxiety therapists have actually welcomed the tapes and use them to reflect on the session, often identifying subtle enactments that they had not been consciously aware of at the time.

The inclusion of outcome monitoring into routine practice makes pragmatic sense because DIT is then comparable with other psychological interventions in a climate of evidence-based practice where lack of evidence is often erroneously construed as evidence of ineffectiveness. As importantly, provided the measures are meaningful to the changes DIT is trying to support, continuous monitoring also serves to focus both patient and therapist on how the work is progressing. If scores remain static, or indeed worsen, over the course of the therapy this can helpfully raise the question of why this is happening. A deterioration in scores on questionnaires should never be taken as absolute evidence that the therapy is failing, but neither can it be dismissed as irrelevant to what is transpiring between the therapist and patient. It should at the very least give pause for thought and lead to a review of what may not feel, and may indeed not be, helpful to the patient.

In DIT, therapists are encouraged to administer measures at the start of each session. Although we recognize that this practice may be felt to be intrusive to the therapeutic process (and sometimes may turn out to be so with some patients), experience bears out that this is typically an intrusion felt more acutely by the therapist than the patient.

In practice, filling in the forms takes up the first few minutes of every session, and can feel awkward as we sit and observe the patient filling in the forms. It is important, however, to not split off the questionnaires from the interaction with the therapist by asking the patient to fill them in before coming in. Integrating this activity within the therapy hour ensures that the therapist can monitor and respond to the patient's communication through the questionnaires. Indeed, once the therapist is acculturated to the routine of outcome monitoring, the "use" made of the questionnaires by the patient becomes grist to the therapeutic mill. For example, one patient reported significant improvement in the sessions, yet her scores on the questionnaires remained very high. When this discrepancy was taken up by the therapist it made it possible to understand at the level of the transference the patient's wish to "punish" the therapist and deprive her of evidence she might share with others that the therapy was of help—an enactment of the grievance the patient harbored towards her mother.

During training DIT sessions are also taped and listened to by the supervisor. As with outcome monitoring, this practice can at first feel threatening to the clinician. The impact it may have on the patient is not infrequently cited as the reason for not taping. In our experience very few patients refuse to be taped or find this intrusive, though the meaning of being taped is invariably worthy of exploration. Some patients regard it an expression of their "specialness" while others may at times fear that what is on tape may be heard by others who would be critical of the patient. The patient's fantasies about being taped always warrant the therapist's acknowledgment, interest, and exploration with the patient.

From the therapist's point of view we have found that once the initial anxiety about taping is overcome, access to the tape is experienced as helpful in reviewing their work. Not uncommonly, as the tape is replayed, the therapist notices a particular quality in the exchange that had not been apparent or consciously registered at the time—in other words, the tape itself functions as an adjunct to supervision even before the supervisor has listened to it and made comments.

Chapter 5

The Interpersonal-Affective Focus

Arriving at a psychodynamic formulation, and explicitly sharing this with the patient in order to negotiate the focus of the work, represents the final outcome of the initial phase. As we saw in the previous chapter a core strategy in the initial phase involves identifying interpersonal and affective patterns in the patient's past and current relationships so as to formulate a recurring configuration of "self" and "other" representations that will become the focus for the remainder of the therapy. In this chapter we will describe how we formulate in DIT so as to arrive at a focus for the therapy. It is this focus that will orient both therapist and patient in the *middle phase* sessions ensuring that some meaningful work and change can be achieved within the time limit.

What is a psychodynamic formulation?

A formulation bridges theory and practice. It ensures that therapy is mapped to the needs of the individual patient and provides a focus for the work. The formulation will thus also inform the direction and goals of treatment.

In a general sense a psychodynamic formulation strives to identify both the external and the internal factors that have contributed to and/or are maintaining the problem. This formulation is a provisional *hypothesis*, which will most likely be refined in collaboration with the patient as the work progresses. It is all too easy to become attached to our hypotheses, but it is incumbent on us to monitor whether we become so married to our hypothesis that we no longer remain alert to what the patient may be trying to communicate that is incongruent with it.

Because it is explicitly shared with the patient, the formulation gives him a chance to respond to it and to work with the therapist to refine it so that there is a good fit between the formulation and the patient's current difficulties. This process is important because if it makes sense to the patient he is more likely to be engaged with the therapy.

The choice of framework for formulating is a question of personal preference, which invariably reflects one's own theoretical allegiances. This is true of DIT, but besides our own theoretical preferences, we also wanted the framework for formulation to be as simple as possible whilst doing justice to the complexity of an individual's mental life. This is why we opted for the IPAF, to which we will now turn.

The interpersonal-affective focus (IPAF): an overview

By session 4 the therapist will have elicited several INs and sketched out the patient's interpersonal map. She will also have identified the relational anxiety embedded in the "cautionary tale." Taken together these sources of information help the therapist to formulate the IPAF, that is, the dominant internal relationship that is linked to the manifest problem.

Our starting point for formulating in DIT is that to understand how the patient relates to others, we have to gain a detailed picture of his internal world of relationships and of the states of mind that this internal world of loving and hating figures—and of loved and hated figures—gives rise to. The internal world, as we conceptualize it in DIT, consists of prototypic schemas involving invariant dimensions of early affectively charged relationships (e.g. experiences of union and separation). In early life, heightened affective exchanges are psychically organizing: they allow the baby to categorize and expect similar experiences. For example, a "negative" experience may be internalized as a working model of an "ugly"-self-relating-to-a humiliating-other. Once learnt, a relational working model sets a template for interpreting later events in a similar way; that is, it generalizes.

External relationships at any stage of the life cycle may then trigger the affects associated with particular relationship constellations and the associated relational fantasy (e.g. "If I get close to another person they will see my ugly self and humiliate me, so it's best to keep to myself"). These mental representations of "self-affectively-interacting-with-other" therefore contain both conscious and nonconscious cognitive and affective components deriving from significant inter-personal experiences with key attachment figures. Although the experiences that contributed to these schemas remain for the most part inaccessible to conscious memory, they nevertheless structure how we think and feel about ourselves and about others. This is why, even though we may not be able to recall early events, we nevertheless continue to organize the present according to developmental models.

In our view a useful way of formulating these dominant internal relationships is found in Kernberg's (1985) distinctive integration of object-relations theory and ego psychology, which focuses on proto-types of positive and negative relationships that become internalized. Following on from this, we conceptualize unconscious conflict as resulting from a clash between particular self and other representa-tions (Kernberg, 1985), resulting in a recurring interpersonal pattern and expectation of others. The IPAF thus consists of four dimensions (see Figure 5.1):

♦ A self-representation (e.g. a demanding infant: "I always ask for too much").

♦ An object-representation (e.g. a rejecting mother: "No-one is there for me when I need them").

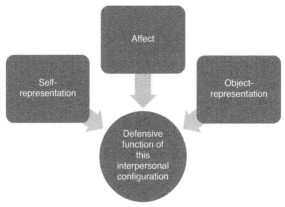

Figure 5.1 IPAF dimensions.

◆ An affect linking the two (e.g. terror: "The worst moments are when I feel in pain and there is no-one to turn to").

◆ The defensive function of this configuration (e.g. avoidance of own aggression—by maintaining the other in one's mind as "always rejecting," the patient can remain in the victim position and avoids reflecting on his own tendency to reject).

The patient's experience of the IPAF

To begin with the description of the self and other representation is just that: a *description* that aims to capture the quality of the patient's experience of himself when he relates, in his mind, to an other to whom particular qualities have been rightly or wrongly attributed. Typically the patient finds this kind of conceptualization relatively unthreatening as it describes his experience without any suggestion of the part he may also play in keeping alive this version of reality. The latter is for the most part the work of the middle phase when the IPAF is "unpacked" and its various nuances and defensive dimensions are explored. Not uncommonly the affect that is identified at this early stage is conscious affect. It is only as the IPAF is worked on that the unconscious affect that is defended against is gradually brought to the patient's conscious attention (e.g. panic that defends against rage).

In our experience of practicing DIT and of supervising our colleagues we have been repeatedly struck by the powerful impact that the articulation of the IPAF has on the patient. Often the patient is deeply affected as he listens to the therapist offering an account of how she has understood his experience. When the IPAF has face validity, and this can be illustrated to the patient through examples of how this pattern is manifest across different domains of his life (e.g. in intimate and work relationships), and how it is also connected with the onset of symptoms, this can help the patient to feel that there is some underlying "sense" to his predicament.

Of course, for some patients, being understood is not a straightforward experience, however benign the therapist's intentions. It may instead feel very exposing or humiliating, as if "caught out." This is especially so because implicit in the IPAF is also an invitation to the patient to consider his role in his predicament. For most patients the

challenge arises when the defensive function of the self–other configuration is added to this description of the "internal state of affairs," as
it were. This is because now the patient is invited to take some responsibility for also "doing" something to his objects: for example, the way
a patient may have a particular investment in seeing himself as someone who is forever being disappointed. In other words, the therapist
attends to the role of the defensive function in maintaining the patient's
psychic equilibrium.

In the middle phase of the work (see Chapter 6) the way in which
the self may also identify with the object becomes more apparent. The
patient may enact a role reversal such that, if we stay with the example
above of an "ugly self" felt to be relating to a "humiliating other," the
patient may, in turn, become the humiliating other in his relationships, locating in someone else the pain of being the undesirable
one—not infrequently locating it in the therapist through a process of
projective identification. The therapist's task then becomes that of
helping the patient to consider his investment in maintaining the
internal status quo, sensitively pointing out its apparent benefits alongside the heavy interpersonal costs and symptomatic expressions.

Inviting the patient to consider the ways in which he may be contributing to his difficulties in this way is more or less easy depending
on how capable the patient is of reflecting on his experience and the
impact *he* may have on other people in his life. For this reason we suggest that the comprehensiveness of the IPAF that is shared with the
patient at session 4 is guided by what the patient appears capable of
taking in at that point, and is accordingly titrated in terms of its content so as to ensure that the patient is not unduly persecuted by it.

It is not uncommon for the defensive function of the IPAF, and the
unconscious affect that links the self–other representation, to be
addressed only in later sessions. By then the patient will have hopefully developed a solid working alliance with the therapist and will
have been helped sufficiently to develop a mentalizing stance such
that he is better equipped to now reflect on his contribution to the
relational impasse captured in the IPAF and how this is connected to
his presenting difficulties.

The therapist needs to be receptive to the patient's conscious and
unconscious experience when hearing the IPAF for the first time so as

to tease out the multilayered nature of his experience of being understood or of realizing how much he has actively, albeit unconsciously, participated in the creation or maintenance of his difficulties.

Case example

Carol, a twenty-seven-year-old woman, was referred because of panic attacks and eating problems, which consisted of erratic bingeing but without vomiting. She binged as a way, as she put it, "of shutting down my feelings." It was only when she ate that she felt like "nothing matters." Her depression had worsened after the break-up of a relationship six months previously. Since then she had felt very worried about the future, fearing that her life was going nowhere. She said that she felt very lonely. She added that she feared loneliness the most.

As the therapist explored her relationships it soon became clear that Carol found it difficult to sustain relationships; she felt that people were often trying to get away from her and she had been told by friends and a previous partner that she could be "too much." She feared this was true. If she was in a relationship she recognized her heightened sensitivity to feeling easily rejected, for example, if friends did not *always* invite her to join them. When with her boyfriend she called him several times a day and would worry if she could not get hold of him.

Carol described a close, yet anxious, attachment to her mother whom she praised for her commitment to charity work and emotional resilience. Her father had died when she was very young. She described her mother as coping very well with raising her as a single parent. As Carol got older, her mother developed a very successful business and worked long hours.

In the first session the therapist experienced Carol as anxious to rapidly establish a closeness with her. Prior to the initial session Carol had phoned several times to confirm that she was coming. The therapist was struck by this behavior and thought that it communicated Carol's anxiety about whether she was kept in mind, but also gave the therapist a more direct experience of how controlling she could be.

In the first session the therapist invited her to think about why she had sought help. Carol had had some prior therapy whilst at university; she had been told then about intensive therapy and wondered whether she should come several times per week because she recognized that her problems were severely restricting her life. The therapist was struck by what she experienced as Carol's over-eagerness to come into therapy, to have sessions all the time, as if she could not bear to be left alone with any gaps when she might have thoughts that could be too disturbing.

To begin with Carol described her mother as a very self-sufficient woman whom she admired greatly. She had berated herself by comparison because she could not "get her act together" like her mother had done after her father died. In the second session Carol spoke some more about her mother. She said that she had missed her mother a great deal as she was growing up. The woman that the week before had been presented as the perfect role model now took on a qualitatively different coloring: her mother was now described as unavailable, at times even selfishly pursuing her own career. When the therapist asked her how she had managed when her mother was away, Carol replied that she did not think about her any more and she just got on with her life.

The therapist tracked this sequence to get a picture of what would happen when the mother came home: Carol said that at first she felt distanced from her and could be quite rejecting of her, but it was not long before she reconnected with her longing for her. She would then turn to her mother for comfort, but only to feel dismissed by her (her mother, for example, would tell her not to cry and she recalled her "physical coldness"). At least this was how she experienced it consciously: it became apparent over the ensuing sessions that Carol could be rather unforgiving and hostile towards others if they were not available to her when she needed them and yet she struggled to see how punishing she could be of them. The therapist therefore wondered about the unconscious investment in keeping the other as "rejecting" as a defense against knowing about her own aggression.

On the basis of this additional information about Carol's experience of her relationship with her mother, the therapist began to formulate that one significant internalized object relationship might be as follows: a needy, deprived self relating to a dismissive, unavailable other. The conscious affect associated with this was, in fact, a lack of affect: Carol described dissociating herself from her feelings, retreating into a "nothing matters" state that she recreated in her binges. However, she had also told the therapist that what she feared most was "loneliness." The therapist hypothesized that the defended-against feeling was that of loneliness and even panic, which she managed by then retreating into binges. This was not an unconscious affect since Carol knew this is what she sometimes felt: what she was not aware of was how she used bingeing as a defense against this internal state of mind (see Figure 5.2).

This formulation could then be applied to the emerging transference and Carol's wish for a very intensive therapy—a theme to which she returned several times in the first few sessions and the therapist felt under pressure to respond. This wish suggested that in coming into therapy the internal model that was activated was one where Carol felt like a very needy, deprived child who needed to secure as many sessions as possible with her therapist as a way of controlling her because she anticipated in her mind an unavailable mother/therapist.

Constructing a formulation: a step-by-step guide

A DIT formulation has several components:

◆ It describes the problem as seen by the patient.

◆ It contextualizes the problem in a developmental framework taking into account temperamental dispositions, physical givens,

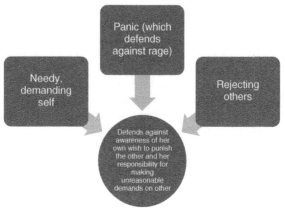

Figure 5.2 Carol's IPAF.

traumatic experiences/life events, past and present relationships, and sociocultural factors.

+ It pulls together this information into an account that meaningfully links the patient's difficulties with a psychological, dynamic process.

Using the psychodynamic formulation aide-mémoire in Box 5.1 let us return to Carol and formulate her problems using this model.

Step 1: Describe the problem

Carol presents with panic and bulimic symptomatology. She uses eating, according to her, as a way of not feeling anything. She also describes relationships problems: she fears that she is not kept in mind and seeks constant reassurance from others.

Step 2: Describe the psychic cost of the problem

Carol acknowledges that she has problems in establishing relation-ships and that she can be suffocating. This alienates others and makes her feel lonely.

Step 3: Contextualize the problem

Carol reports a difficult early life. Her father died when she was very young and she subsequently lived with her mother. Her mother was a

Box 5.1 DIT formulation aide-mémoire

Step 1: Describe the problem

Ask yourself: How does the patient view the problem: what or who is the patient reacting to?

Step 2: Describe the cost of the problem

Ask yourself: What limitations in the patient's functioning or distortions in his perception of others and self have resulted from the problem?

Step 3: Contextualize the problem. Identify relevant predisposing factors and current external factors (e.g. unemployment) that are relevant to understanding the onset and course of the symptoms/difficulties

Ask yourself: How do the environmental (e.g. history of trauma, developmental factors influencing processing of trauma, family system, other relevant life events) and/or biological givens (e.g. disability) relate to the presenting problem?

Step 4: Describe the patient's recurrent self–other representation that is meaningfully connected to the presenting symptoms/difficulties

Ask yourself: How does the patient experience himself in relationship to others?

- Identify who does what to whom and the associated affect
- How is this internalized object relationship manifest in the patient's current life?
- How might the representations of self/others influence and be influenced by current relationships?
- How do these internalized object relationships manifest themselves in the relationship with you?

Step 5: Identify the defensive function of the identified self–other representation

Ask yourself: What is the patient afraid of/trying to avoid in himself? What are the possible consequences of change?

single parent and a busy professional woman who had to leave Carol in the care of nannies. Carol therefore often felt lonely, longing for her mother's return, but then resenting her mother, and needing to punish her when she returned.

She describes her mother telling her not to cry. Carol thus learnt early on that the best way to manage her affects was to switch herself off from them, so that she did not have to feel her mother's absence and her loneliness.

In her adult life, Carol encounters more loneliness because she appears incapable of establishing an intimacy without taking over the other person in an attempt to control an object whose attention she internally fears she cannot sustain.

Step 4: Describe the recurring object-relationship that is meaningfully connected to the onset and/or maintenance of symptoms and the affect that is linked with the activation of the pattern

Carol experiences herself as easily rejected. She needs constant reassurance in her relationships because she does not trust that she is kept in mind. She experiences the other as unavailable to her such that she has to chase the other, as with her partners whom she phones several times a day, to concretely reinforce her presence in their mind. In the assessment relationship these patterns manifest themselves in her need to confirm the time of her appointment and in her wish to have intensive therapy as if anything less would expose her to the experience of not being kept in mind (i.e., that another patient will replace her in the therapist's mind). The perceived loss of the object's undivided attention elicits overwhelming anxiety in the form of panic attacks.

Step 5: Identify the defensive function of the recurring pattern

Carol's experience of her self as needy and demanding and of the object as rejecting is not a pleasurable one—it causes her significant levels of distress. Yet to relinquish this version of reality would also mean having to face her own rage towards the object and to not only her tendency control the object (of which she had some awareness), but also her wish to punish the object, and hence she would have to take responsibility for her own aggression.

The trial interpretation: working towards sharing the IPAF

In the initial sessions the therapist will make a trial interpretation both to elaborate the evolving formulation in light of the patient's response to the interpretation, and to assess the patient's capacity to make use of such interventions. If we return to Carol, before sharing a possible IPAF, in session 3 the therapist took up the interpersonal pattern in the transference. The therapist proceeded gradually, mindful that Carol was highly sensitive to feeling criticized and "pushed out" by the other, so here she raised the less contentious "rejecting other" pole of the experience (not her self-representation as demanding):

> You have mentioned several times your sense that what you need is an intensive therapy. You may well be right about that. I don't yet have a clear view of that myself, but what I have been thinking as we talk together is that you are very anxious about starting this therapy and you may be worried about whether I will be available to you when you need me to be, about whether I will keep you in mind when we are not meeting. Wanting more sessions may be your way of ensuring that you are firmly in my mind and that no-one else can take up your place in my mind.

Carol was silent and then started to cry. She recognized that this was what she always did in her relationships: she couldn't bear to not be "central" to the other person. Carol's response to the transference interpretation gave the therapist the confidence to share the emerging IPAF and to engage Carol in refining it. The therapist shared the IPAF along these lines:

> One of the things that I have been really struck by over the last four sessions is that you seem to be very preoccupied with whether, as you put it, you are "central" to the people you want to be close to, with whether they keep you in mind. It's been the case here too, between us, with you feeling very worried that unless you book yourself in to see me several times a week you will drop out of my mind and you will find yourself on your own—an experience that is familiar and terrifying for you. It seems to me that as you approach a relationship you typically feel yourself to be very needy, demanding even, and expect the other to be unavailable to you. You are terrified of being left on your own and so you try to find ways of minimizing the likelihood of this

happening and, as you helpfully recognize, this can paradoxically have the opposite effect to the one you are hoping for: the other person may feel controlled and then they may pull away. And then this only confirms your worst fears and the cycle begins again.

Put this way, the patient and therapist could then return to the IPAF when exploring particular INs in the course of therapy, inviting the patient to stand back from her immediate experience and engaging her in thinking about this pattern.

Using the patient's language and metaphors

When formulating and constructing the IPAF it is very helpful to personalize it so as to capture the patient's immediate, affective experience. This requires paying careful attention to the patient's choice of words, the imagery associated with his descriptions of feeling states, or the metaphors used. The therapist's attunement to these idiosyncratic terms often also serves to convey to the patient that she has listened carefully.

There can be a significant affective gap between describing the self, for example, as "unattractive", and using the patient's more idiosyncratic self-descriptor, which often carries greater valence in the internal world, as in the example below. Particular words or expressions then become shared markers for the recognition of the self and/or other representations.

Case example

Timothy, a thirty-year-old man, was referred for help with recurrent depression. He presented as likeable and eager to please. He was the youngest of ten children and said he was severely bullied by elder brothers. He described himself as "crafty" and told the therapist stories of conning or reacting aggressively to others. And yet he also described feeling "like a loser."

In session 3, the therapist formulated an IPAF that proposed Timothy's self-representation as "a loser" in relation to an object who treats him badly/humiliates him. This particular configuration left him feeling humiliated and aroused in him a need to seek revenge, triumphing over others through various forms of "crafty" behavior so as to reverse the representation of self and other and to thereby triumph over the felt-to-be-humiliating object. This included the development of a false self—a "Jack the lad," cheerful chap persona—and the denial of more vulnerable, sensitive aspects of self. The overarching impact of all his defensive strategies was to keep the object at a distance and to be responsible for repeatedly losing potentially enriching interpersonal experiences.

Timothy found the IPAF helpful and agreed to work on this focus. The earlier part of the middle phase sessions with Timothy focused upon the mechanisms by which he kept the object at a distance and, indeed, kept his "true" (more vulnerable, pained) self at a distance via a "false" pleasing, "cheeky chappy" presentation. He and the therapist noticed his rivalrous relationship with others—his need to be the favorite and most liked, but how this presentation belied more real feelings of being left out and vulnerable. This experience was presented as making sense in view of his being one of 10 children, vying for parental attention, but emphasis was placed on the fact that his strategies for coping with this had now become problematic for him. It was then possible to look at the ways in which he attempted to triumph over others as a way of managing a very painful sense of himself as "a loser."

For some time the therapist struggled to take anything up in the transference. In thinking about this the therapist became aware that Timothy's interpersonal strategies of keeping others away from his vulnerable, "true" self were very seductive and compelling. The therapist had to work hard not to be pulled into his central self–other dynamic and to thus maintain her ability to think—to notice his avoidance of "real" feeling and his manipulation of the truth. The therapist had to stand back from the way in which he used somewhat glib, emotionally flat, or clichéd reporting of the week's events to keep her at a distance from the more painful feelings that he was unable to bear. This involved managing her own countertransference to not be overwhelmed, confused, irritated, or made to feel "mad" by the manner in which his accounts became elusive and slippery as a result of his providing her with slightly differing facts and emphasis at different points.

Using the experience in the transference the therapist was able to make more productive inroads into reaching Timothy and helping him to make sense of the INs he was bringing. Earlier narratives of rivalry, his own "craftiness", and being treated badly began to be replaced by ones of loneliness and isolation.

In the middle stages of the work with Timothy, he began many sessions recounting how "lonely" he felt. Of course, this had a meaning within the session, as well as beyond, and enabled useful work around his desire for closeness with the therapist, combined with his ways of avoiding this. In the later middle part of the work, Timothy was more able to grasp his avoidance of emotional relating and the ways in which his more narcissistic "best beloved" requirements interfered with this. As Timothy became more in touch with his own pain, vulnerability, and need, he was able in a more real way to focus on his need to triumph over others, often in quite aggressive and destructive ways. Earlier in the work he could see the impact of such behavior on himself, but in the later stages he was also able to feel some shame and to acknowledge the impact of devious or aggressive behavior on others.

In the middle to end stages of work with Timothy, the therapist together with Timothy was able to productively utilize some of the quippy phrases that he used in the earlier stages to distance her and himself from his emotions. Particularly useful was a throw-away phrase he brought into an early session—DTA (don't trust anybody)—and his initially proud descriptions of himself as "Jack the lad" and "the golden boy." In a more painful, but very punitive and persecutory moment, he also described himself as a "honeymonster." All of these phrases became invaluable to the work, as they were used as signifiers of the central, identified interpersonal dynamic.

The ending phase of work was defined by sadder feelings and a sense of mourning for the more "real" self that he has so effectively denied. He was able to manage working with some of his frustrated feelings about ending and his fear of, combined with an excitement about, a referral for longer-term group work.

Using the transference and countertransference to inform the formulation

Three sources of information are available to assist us in the process of formulating self–object representations: the patient's narrative account of his childhood history with significant others, the patient's current relationships, and the relationship the patient develops with us. To arrive at an IPAF the therapist actively draws not just on the content of the patient's narratives, but also on the experience and observation of the patient's ways of relating within the session.

The transference is what makes it possible for us to be drawn into the patient's world so that we may experience it ourselves rather than relying on the patient's report of his relationships. For Freud the transference was a form of remembering, but, as Lear puts it, this is a highly particular kind of remembering, moreover one that:

> is not a form of recollection, but of memorialisation, an enactment designed to make the present into an artefact of the past . . . The aim of the enactment is to endow the world with comprehensible meaning (1993: 745).

Here Lear highlights two very important functions of the transference: the way in which it creates a familiar, "known" (at an unconscious level) road map for how to relate and what to expect from others, and how this map performs a vital function in the patient's internal world. This is why the therapist can often reliably anticipate the patient's fierce investment in keeping alive the unconscious pattern that is also part of the problem.

The therapist makes use of her understanding of the transference and countertransference to develop hypotheses about problematic interpersonal patterns. At this early stage transference interpretations are kept to a minimum, but the therapist's understanding of the developing transference is central in helping her to generate hypotheses about the patient's interpersonal functioning.

Not all patients are overly preoccupied in an obtrusive manner with the therapist at the very outset, hence the transference may be less obvious and/or intrusive with some. For others, however, the anxieties about starting therapy are acute. If the patient presents, from the outset, as very preoccupied with the therapist, which is more likely if there is a comorbid PD, the therapist engages the patient in elaborating a description of what preoccupies him about the therapist and about what he is feeling.

Case example

Ms A., who was referred for social anxiety and mild depression, arrived for the first session apparently very anxious, and found it hard to speak. The therapist noted that the patient could barely establish eye contact and that she looked noticeably stiff in her posture whilst the therapist set out the boundaries for the initial consultation.

The therapist asked Ms A. how she was feeling, to which Ms A. replied that she had not wanted to come and had only come because her GP had sent her. The therapist invited Ms A. to tell her a bit about how the consultation with the GP had gone. The patient spoke about how she had felt that the GP dismissed her problems, and with conviction she added that the GP thought that she was to blame. The therapist enquired about what it was that had made her feel so sure that this was what the GP believed. The patient said that the GP was rushed in her manner and had barely asked her any questions, and that she looked disapproving.

Having explored this exchange, focusing in particular on what the patient was feeling and thinking, and what she imagined the GP was feeling and thinking, the therapist abstracted the underlying relational pattern and acknowledged that she had felt both neglected and disapproved of, and asked Ms A. whether this was a familiar feeling for her. The patient replied that people were not interested in her, and that she often felt looked down on by others. The therapist then linked this to how the patient had started the session feeling anxious, and that perhaps she was now worried about what the therapist was thinking about her. The patient replied that when the therapist had described what was going to happen, and that they had only fifty minutes, this had made her feel that the therapist was just going through the motions, that she was not really interested. The therapist said that this seemed to be a familiar experience, just like with the GP. The patient agreed. The therapist tentatively added that the patient seemed to expect that others would be dismissive of her and that, from this perspective, the therapist stating the length of the session no longer felt like a fact that she might or might not like, but instead she heard it as a confirmation that the therapist was simply not interested in her. The therapist added that if this is how she felt, then she could understand why the patient was finding it hard to open up.

The intervention illustrated in the case example is characteristic of how the DIT therapist engages with an interpersonal scenario and illustrates of some of the key features of a DIT transference interpretation in these early sessions:

- It deconstructs an IN (the story about the GP) in order to abstract an implicit relational pattern.
- It links this pattern to the here-and-now relationship with the therapist.
- It frames it in the context of current triggers (starting therapy).
- It validates the patient's experience and conveys that her response is understandable given the version of self and other that has been activated.

How to select a focus

By the third or fourth session, the therapist will have a working hypothesis about the most salient IPAF that is meaningfully connected to the symptoms. The formulation of the most relevant IPAF is probably the most challenging juncture for the therapist, not least because patients will present with a number of interpersonal patterns that are more or less adaptive and which reflect particular qualities of self and other representations. The therapist therefore has to decide between a number of relational constellations to arrive at the most productive route through which to understand, and work on, the patient's current difficulties.

In selecting a focus we are looking for a *specific* interpersonal constellation that sheds some light on the onset and/or maintenance of the symptoms/difficulties. Here the time line of the symptoms is helpful since we are trying to distil what pattern was activated in the patient's mind around the time of the onset of symptoms.

In practice the descriptors of the self–other poles of the IPAF need to be specific and distinct. For example, during the initial sessions one therapist was able to identify with the patient that he often felt

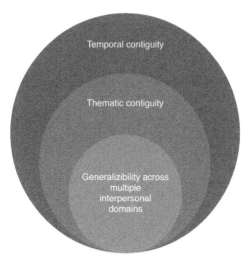

Figure 5.3 Criteria for selecting an IPAF.

"defective" and "a burden." Alongside this they established together that other people were frequently experienced as "critical, patronizing, and unpredictable." In order to arrive at an IPAF the therapist had to do more work since "being defective" and "being a burden" are not the same experiences. It was possible that the patient's self-representation as "defective" exposed him to the experience of feeling that he was a burden, which is quite different to a self-representation as "being a burden." Similarly, there are potentially significant differences between an object experienced as critical/patronizing and one felt to be "unpredictable." Faced with this not uncommon potential multitude of possible self–other constellations, in order to select a focus, the therapist is guided by three considerations (see Figure 5.3):

◆ The connection between the IPAF and the presenting symptoms needs to be meaningful and have face validity for the patient (i.e., temporal contiguity).

◆ The validity of the IPAF is supported by a goodness of fit with the patient's patterns as evident through the INs (i.e., thematic contiguity).

◆ The IPAF is recurring and manifest across a number of the patient's relationships (i.e., its generalizability across multiple interpersonal domains).

Sharing the IPAF with the patient

Once the therapist has developed some ideas about the IPAF these are shared with the patient in a tentative manner that clearly communicates the therapist's interest in the patient's own views about it. For example the therapist might say:

> Having listened to what you have told me over the last few sessions about how you are feeling and what you are most concerned about in your life right now, I have some ideas about what's been going on for you and how this might help us to make sense of the symptoms that have brought you here. I would like to share these with you to see what you think so that we can see whether this might be of help in finding a focus for our work.

The therapist can then present the patient with an account of how his difficulties have developed, the relational pattern that appears to be connected with their onset and/or maintenance, and the impact this has on current relationships.

Throughout this process the therapist is alert to the patient's response to the formulation in order to ascertain its relevance and/or perceived threat to his equilibrium. This is very important because, as we noted earlier, the IPAF describes an interpersonal pattern that as well as being distressing to the patient (i.e., it is ego-dystonic) may nevertheless serve a protective function and therefore may be felt to be psychically necessary.

The aim is to work *collaboratively* with the patient to promote a sense of agency and participation in arriving at a formulation that is meaningful to him. In one sense all psychodynamic approaches, at their best, are collaborative. In DIT we use this term not only as a reminder of this important feature of the therapeutic encounter, but also to underline that the DIT therapist is *explicitly* collaborative in so far as she actively seeks out the patient's view of the formulation and engages him in refining it.

It is very important to approach the task of formulating in an open, tentative manner that invites the patient to comment and express any anxieties or disagreement he has about the suggested focus. The discussion of the IPAF should provide the patient with an opportunity to ask questions and to clarify and agree therapeutic aims so that he feels engaged with the work. A formulation is a working hypothesis and, as such, requires regular revision in light of patient feedback and the therapist's evolving understanding of the patient over time.

A frequent question posed by therapists learning the model is what they should do if the patient disagrees with the IPAF. If the therapist has actively engaged the patient in developing the IPAF, if it meets the three criteria listed above (thematic contiguity, temporal contiguity, and generalizability), and if the therapist has been responsive to the patient's feedback, it is very unusual for the IPAF to become a source of conflict and disagreement because it is the outcome of the patient's and the therapist's joint efforts. The IPAF, as we have seen, may feel very challenging and the patient may struggle to work on it during the middle phase, but in our experience this kind of natural resistance to taking responsibility for what we do to ourselves and to our objects is far more common than disagreements over the actual content of the IPAF.

Case example

Marc is in his mid-twenties—a rather small man, studious-looking, with an intense frown that had a peculiarly distancing effect on the therapist on first meeting him.

His GP referred him after having signed him off work for two consecutive weeks due to stress, following a difficulty with his boss. Marc had been in this job for just under a year when he started to feel bullied by his boss.

Marc is the eldest of two. His father died unexpectedly of a heart attack when he was five years old. Following his death, his mother appeared to have sunk into a very depressed state of mind from which she never fully emerged. Marc still lives at home with his mother while his younger brother left home to move in with his girlfriend just under a year ago.

Marc presents as rather subdued, and on first meeting him the therapist found it hard to engage him. She felt that he was depressed and his social withdrawal was marked. As he described his relationships, he conveyed a sense that he was always on guard, as if he could never quite let himself relax. He was very anxious in the first session.

Marc explained that he had never taken to his boss because he was "loud" and "brash." A few months prior to being signed off work by his GP, Marc had felt particularly humiliated by his boss after he was openly critical of one of Marc's reports in front of other colleagues. At the time, Marc had barely spoken, feeling himself immediately to be "stupid," and he felt that he had not defended his position. Subsequently, he felt that everyone viewed him differently and he found it increasingly hard to even look people in the eye when he was at work. He ruminated over this exchange in his mind and the more he did so the more angry he became. He spoke about the "injustice" of it all as he was hardworking and diligent.

As Marc spoke about his difficulties, the therapist became aware that he was having a particular impact on her: she felt she was being recruited into siding with Marc against the boss who had become the personification of evil. The therapist made a mental note of this, but said nothing at this stage. This feeling nevertheless grew stronger as he described in more detail his relationship with his younger brother. He felt that his brother had acted selfishly, leaving home just when Marc had taken up a new job and their mother had become more severely depressed. Consequently, Marc had felt that the burden of care for his mother had fallen on him, as he felt it had always done since his father's death.

The description of his brother bore an uncanny similarity to Marc's hated boss. His brother was described as loud, unthinking, and selfish. They had never been close, and he reluctantly acknowledged that his brother was very successful in life. He spontaneously recounted that as they were only eighteen months apart, they shared many friends together and went to the same school, but that he felt he was always in his shadow because of his more outgoing personality. When the therapist invited him to elaborate on this Marc gave a very detailed account of his brother's superior physical achievements. In this respect he thought that his brother had taken after their father who had been an excellent runner in his time. He added somewhat pointedly that his brother had been fortunate to inherit his father's height and strength whereas he had followed in the maternal footsteps: his mother's family was described as a family of "clever thinkers prone to depression."

Marc's current interpersonal world was very impoverished and had been so for many years, not simply since he became more evidently depressed. He had one close male friend who struck the therapist as also quite a fragile, anxious individual. Nevertheless they did meet every few weeks and shared an interest in film.

Marc had not had any girlfriends in the last five years. The only relationship of note had lasted a few months. He had met his then girlfriend when he had just started university. The relationship ended unhappily when the girlfriend complained that he never wanted to go out. Marc justified this in terms of prioritizing his studies at the time because he wanted to get a good degree.

The therapist enquired about how Marc had felt when his brother left home to live with his girlfriend. He replied dismissively that he did not care about what his brother did with his life, but that he certainly would never choose a girl like his brother had done. He described the girlfriend as an "airhead" who enjoyed clubbing and clothes.

The therapist spent some time exploring Marc's relationship with his parents. Marc said he did not really feel that he knew his father except through his mother's rose-tinted glasses. He had grown up hearing what an impressive character he had been, and he mentioned twice the way his mother referred to the father's "stature" both concretely, as he had indeed been tall and strong, and because of his standing in the world of work. As he spoke he conveyed a sense of hopelessness about his own capacity to be impressive, and the therapist reflected this back to him.

By the end of session 2 the therapist had become conscious of a pattern in the room: whenever she tried to be empathic or made some observation, Marc either appeared to ignore it or typically replied that "it was not quite like that." The therapist began to feel that she was being carefully scrutinized and duly criticized, as if in the room the roles had been reversed: it was now Marc who was in some way criticizing her reports, just as he reported his boss had done to him. By now the therapist also hypothesized that Marc had probably always felt second best in relation to both the idealized father figure in his mother's mind and the younger brother who had become his living embodiment.

In session 3 the therapist explored further the circumstances around the time when Marc's brother had left home. It became clear that the onset of a more insidious state of depression dated back to that time, and that it had then been further aggravated by the more recent incident at work. It emerged that the mother had felt bereft by the brother's decision to move away from the family home. She appeared to have been stuck in an unresolved grief reaction following the death of her husband, which was fueled with new impetus by the departure of her younger son. All this appeared to have deeply angered Marc, who had seemingly always felt in the shadow of his father and brother's greater stature in his mother's eyes. The incident at work had been the final blow for him as he had somehow always managed to reassure himself of his superior intellect as a defense against his deep-rooted conviction that he was simply not good enough for his mother. To be attacked publicly, as he saw it, for producing a bad report reduced his intellectual stature and he felt profoundly humiliated and exposed to the critical eyes of others. His anxiety indeed had a distinctly paranoid flavor. His basic response to this interpersonal scenario was one of passive aggression, where he said nothing, withdrew into himself, and internally remained locked in a grievance against the other person. His most profound grievance was towards the parental couple in his mind by whom he felt painfully excluded.

In approaching a possible focus, the therapist began by summarizing the way in which Marc had conveyed to her his long-standing experience of not having any stature in his mother's eyes, and that this characterized more generally his expectation of how other people viewed him. She acknowledged the importance to him of his intellectual pursuits as a way of reassuring himself and others that he did have substance and stature in his own right. Consequently work had been overvalued such that it had not only pulled him away from developing relationships, but also made him highly sensitive to any slight to his intellect. Marc responded to this partial summary saying that at times he did wonder to himself what the point of life was. Bearing in mind the importance of engagement at this early stage, the therapist reflected on the sense of futility that underpinned Marc's overall presentation, but she also observed that he had nevertheless allowed himself to come for help and that this was positive.

The therapist then elaborated further what she had understood so far and spoke with Marc about the heavy burden of having not just to bear the meaning for him of the early loss of his father, but perhaps even more significantly to have to nurse his mother through her ongoing sense of loss, which he could never assuage. The therapist spoke empathically of how he seemed to feel that he had lived in the shadow of his father and brother, both of whom had managed to escape the fate of the "clever thinkers prone to depression," leaving him feeling as if was forever lagging behind them in some fundamental way, which nothing could change. At the same time he was having to take care of a mother who both needed him and made him feel second best.

Marc seemed to respond positively to this formulation, but the therapist detected some hesitation. He emphasized that in the intellectual domain he had always shone, but that somehow this was never really valued, even though he had always thought that his mother, herself an academic, prized intelligence. The therapist wondered to herself whether this response might be indicative of Marc's experience of feeling in some way criticized by her, but she decided not to intervene along these lines as she did not feel she had enough evidence for this. Rather, she observed that he seemed to have always been very preoccupied with what his mother was looking for, and that he felt confused about what she valued and admired. His whole life in a way had been devoted to getting it right for his mother rather than for himself.

She then wondered with him as to whether now that they were negotiating what to work on in therapy, he might be similarly preoccupied with what he imagined the therapist would prize. This appeared to resonate with Marc, who observed how anxious he had felt each time he had come for the session. He then reported a dream he had had the night before the third session in which he had been jeered at by a group of adolescents. In the dream he wanted to shout back, but no words came out.

By this stage the therapist felt confident enough to propose an IPAF (Figure 5.4). She suggested that a recurring experience for Marc in his relationships was to feel that he was small, lacking in stature, insufficient, while the other person was more typically either explicitly humiliating and rejecting (as he had felt his boss had been recently) or more implicitly humiliating (as he felt his mother had been, leaving him feeling that he could never live up to his father's/brother's stature). His only option seemed to be to follow on in the maternal family tradition of "clever thinkers prone to depression." Distressing though this was, the therapist suggested that this way at least Marc comforted himself with a likeness to his mother, which he felt only he shared with her. Marc was intrigued by this suggestion and told the therapist that as he was growing up what he had most enjoyed were the evenings with his mother when he used to read poetry with her. Although the therapist was moved by this image she also sensed Marc's wish to create an intense exchange with her, which did not feel comfortable. Again at this early stage, the therapist only made a mental note of this, and it would only be interpreted if this developed into a resistance in the course of treatment.

The therapist suggested that although Marc's overt response to the interpersonal scenario in which he feels humiliated was to feel impotent and to typically withdraw (as in the dream, he loses his voice), internally a far more angry conversation took place in which he tried to defend himself. At this stage the therapist did

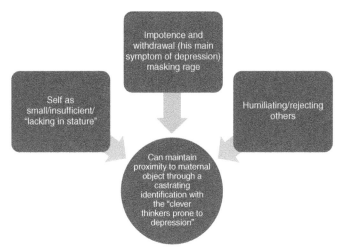

Figure 5.4 Marc's IPAF.

not share her hypothesis that Marc also took up the position of being the critical one in his own mind and subjected the other to harsh scrutiny, because she considered that this would be too much for him to take on board at this point and might indeed make him feel criticized by her. However, this would be an important theme that deserved further elaboration during the course of therapy.

Chapter 6

The Middle Phase

The middle phase of DIT requires both the patient's and the therapist's concentrated effort to stay focused on the agreed IPAF. The therapist works with the patient to identify and understand this dominant, recurring pattern as it plays itself out in current relationships, including the relationship with the therapist, and she highlights its impact on the patient's current functioning and symptoms. In this chapter we will review in more detail the core aims and strategies that guide the *middle phase* (sessions 5–12).

Aims

The overarching aim of the therapist's interventions at this stage in the therapy is to stimulate the patient's capacity to think about and understand his thoughts and feelings, and how these underpin the identified pattern of relating (and its varied behavioral manifestations) that may seem strange or self-defeating. More specifically, the therapist has several aims in mind in approaching the work of the middle phase sessions:

- To help the patient identify areas of difficulty in his relationships that pertain to the IPAF.
- To support his engagement in reflecting on how these difficulties relate to his current symptoms (e.g. how the feelings of panic might relate to the argument with X during the week).
- To help the patient understand his characteristic ways of managing areas of difficulty in his relationships and to point out the "cost" of these strategies, that is, working actively on characteristic defenses.

- To help the patient reflect on his state of mind and the feelings and thoughts he attributes to others in order to highlight the activation and implications of the IPAF.
- To support the patient in trying out new ways of approaching relationship difficulties.

Sequence of movement in middle phase sessions

In DIT each session starts with the patient filling in outcome monitoring data. In this sense it is the therapist who opens every session. The review of the forms provides a focus and entry point into discussing how the patient has been feeling in the intervening week. The patient is invited by the therapist to reflect on how his scores relate to how he has been feeling in the week. A deterioration or improvement in the depression or anxiety scales prompts an exploration of what may have contributed to this.

Besides this structured way of starting the sessions, there is no set agenda to the sessions as such, as in CBT for example, and yet the IPAF *is* the agenda for every session. The therapist always approaches what the patient brings with the IPAF in mind. This is important and somewhat different to the more free-floating attention characteristic of the therapist's approach in open-ended psychodynamic therapy. Having said this, in common with other psychodynamic approaches, the middle phase sessions have a more emergent quality that denotes the therapist's efforts to create a space for unconscious meanings to be elaborated and reflected upon.

Indeed, being focused, whilst precluding attending to all of the patient's dynamics, does not preclude listening to his unconscious communications: in DIT the therapist pays attention to the patient's imaginative life (e.g. conscious and unconscious fantasies, dreams, metaphors) and nonverbal communications (e.g. tone of voice; body posture), and uses these manifestations to deepen the understanding of the patient, and hence as the basis for a more focused interpretation related to the IPAF. Likewise, the therapist allows her own subjective associations and ideas to form in response to the patient's communications and makes use of these to inform her understanding of the patient.

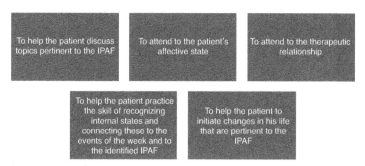

Figure 6.1 Middle phase strategies.

Because sessions in this phase are less structured, it becomes easier for the therapist to wander into more diffuse explorations of the patient's internal world. Here, it is helpful for the therapist to keep in mind the aims of DIT so as to get back to the agreed focus. At the same time, the therapist will need to tolerate a degree of uncertainty and ambiguity when trying to understand the patient's communications so as to not foreclose exploration. Balancing these dual requirements is an important skill that develops with experience of the protocol as the therapist acquires a more direct sense of what it is possible to achieve within one session, and over the course of sixteen sessions, such that she can then pace herself accordingly.

The ability to pace oneself cannot be taught as such—each therapist has to find her own way of navigating through the protocol with enough room for the elaboration and exploration of the patient's experience, but with sufficient focus to ensure the patient can begin to work on an important pattern. Although sixteen sessions may strike some colleagues as impossibly brief, in our experience it is often possible to help patients to make significant changes—or at least to initiate the process of change—within this time limit (Gellman et al., 2010).

The middle phase sessions are gradually structured by the five therapeutic strategies during this phase, as summarized in Figure 6.1. They tend to progress from a more open-ended exploration of what is on the patient's mind at the start of the session as the symptoms are reviewed and/or the preceding week's events, and linking this to the IPAF, on to a more concentrated focus on the patient's state of mind, and finally to engaging the patient in reflecting on how he might

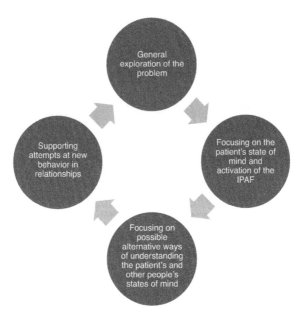

Figure 6.2 Sequence of movement in the middle phase sessions.

handle a problematic situation differently (Figure 6.2). This sequence describes a prototypic session in the middle phase, but it would be unhelpful to view this as cast in stone: in some sessions, for example, there may be little or no possibility for engaging the patient in reflecting on alternative ways of managing how he asserts his needs in a relationship and this may not occur until the following session. It would, however, be very unusual for a middle phase session to make no reference to the IPAF: by and large explicit reference to the IPAF is frequent and consistent in every session in the absence of an acute, immediate crisis, which would of necessity temporarily divert both therapist and patient away from the agreed focus (e.g. an unexpected bereavement).

Tracking the IPAF: eliciting interpersonal narratives (INs) to illustrate the activation of the IPAF

During the middle phase a core strategy is to help the patient to explore the IPAF. This involves assiduously relating the content of interventions to the interpersonal and affective themes that the formulation has identified as the focus of the therapy.

One of the key interventions in this phase is to support the elaboration of INs because it is through these that the IPAF will become apparent. This gives the therapist an opportunity to draw the patient's attention to how it is manifest in his current relationships and how it relates to his presenting symptoms. Connections are made, as appropriate, between current concerns and the IPAF across three interpersonal domains: the therapeutic relationship, current relationships, and past relationships (with less emphasis on the latter).

Some patients struggle to report INs either because they effectively have very few relationships in their current lives or because they want to avoid really thinking about their relationships, preferring instead the relative safety of discussing their problems in abstract terms. When this is the case this will require some redirection back onto a more tangible interpersonal focus. For example, the therapist might say:

> You have a lot of interesting ideas about why you feel as you do and I wonder if you could give me an example of when you felt this way with another person during the last week.

Alternatively, the therapist might consider it more helpful to take up in the transference the patient's retreat into a more cut off, intellectual mode. Either way the strategy is to engage the patient in reflecting on what is actually happening, *now*, in his relationships.

The therapist thus displays curiosity about interpersonal scenarios, asking questions and for clarifications as necessary, to bring into focus an interpersonal exchange so as to highlight a salient repetitive pattern. Whenever the patient presents an IN, as the therapist listens, she is scanning for the following to build a picture in her mind of the patient's internal world, as summarized in Figure 6.3: who is talking/doing what to whom; who feels what towards whom; and how does the therapist feel as she listens.

Through unpacking an IN with the patient the aim is to engage the patient in thinking about what other kinds of conversations might be possible for him and that might be more or less helpful. This may then provide an opportunity for identifying a new way of responding that the patient can be encouraged to try out in between sessions.

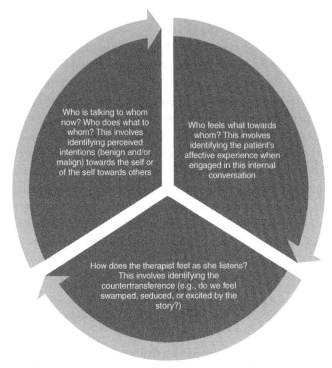

Figure 6.3 Abstracting interpersonal-affective patterns from INs.

Staying focused

However experienced, when learning any new model, we will all have to make some adjustments to our technique that will feel more or less congruent with our known and preferred way of working. Working to a specified focus can feel very difficult at first especially for colleagues accustomed to working long term with open-ended contracts.

Besides the challenge of formulating rather rapidly, and hence of finding a focus for the therapy by (approximately) the fourth session, the other main challenge encountered by DIT practitioners is how to stay focused once a focus has been identified (Box 6.1). Of course we might say that all psychodynamic approaches have a focus in so far as the patient's unconscious mental life is our focus. Indeed, "maintaining a dynamic focus" describes two distinct yet related activities (Lemma et al., 2008). First, it refers to maintaining the primary focus

Box 6.1 Staying focused on the IPAF

It involves:

◆ Helping the patient to identify relevant interpersonal and affective pattern(s) through an exploration of INs and (where relevant) their elaboration in the transference

◆ Helping the patient explore themes relevant to the agreed IPAF through the use of techniques such as clarification, confrontation, and interpretation (see Chapter 7)

◆ Relating the content of interventions to the interpersonal and affective themes pertinent to the IPAF

◆ Helping the patient to identify and explore the meaning of diversions away from the agreed focus (e.g. because it is too painful to address)

on the exploration of the patient's unconscious experience. Essentially this means that all aspects of the work are approached with an analytic attitude. Secondly, it refers to working on a particular dynamic theme or conflict to the relative exclusion of others for the duration of the therapy. This is usually the case in time-limited therapy, as in DIT, where it is essential to negotiate with the patient a circumscribed interpersonal pattern that will provide direction and a boundary for both patient and therapist.

The IPAF is prioritized to the relative exclusion of other possible foci for the duration of the therapy. This is a central challenge shared by all brief approaches, but can present particular challenges for some therapists who may feel that they are short-changing the patient by not addressing a range of unconscious processes that will be apparent to them. Here it is helpful for the therapist to remind herself of the aims of DIT, which, though more modest relative to the aims shared by longer-term psychodynamic therapy, can nevertheless make a tangible, immediate difference to the patient's capacity to function in his day-to-day life.

Deviations from the focus *will* occur, however competent the therapist is. When they do this is a cue for the therapist to think about why this may be happening: is the patient feeling the strain of working on the IPAF? Is it asking too much of the patient? Is the focus felt to be threatening the internal status quo? The task therefore becomes identifying the defensive function of the deviation from the focus.

Where the deviation from the focus occurs because the patient raises other issues that are important to him, but which do not pertain directly to the IPAF, the therapist sensitively acknowledges their importance, but reminds the patient of the agreed focus and the brevity of the treatment, which precludes an in-depth exploration of other areas of his life. If the therapist identifies the need for further therapy, this can be discussed with the patient in the ending phase. Similarly, unexpected life events that occur during the course of the therapy (such as a bereavement) should not go by unacknowledged and responded to in some way. The therapist will need to rely on her tact and sensitivity to guide her in identifying whether the therapy can continue or whether the life event is of such magnitude that the agreed focus becomes less relevant.

Sometimes, however, the patient may keep diverging from the agreed focus simply because the wrong focus was selected. Here, as in any other situation where it becomes clear that the therapist and patient have misunderstood each other, or where there is an impasse in the therapy, the therapist approaches this openly, is receptive to the patient's experience and feedback about what is felt to not be helpful, and strives to engage jointly with the patient in working out a way forwards (see also Chapter 10).

A typical concern that arises for therapists applying this protocol is about becoming very repetitive because the IPAF can seem restrictive in the context of the myriad facets of any individual's internal mental life. In one sense this is true: we are explicitly selecting only one segment of the patient's functioning and there are many others. But the concern about repetitiveness is not one shared by patients who, on the whole, welcome this assiduous emphasis on the IPAF because it helps them to concentrate, over a short period of time, on working on something that can be identified and named in their current functioning, and hopefully modified to some degree. The specificity of the IPAF is, in fact, containing for most patients. By the end of the sixteen sessions it has become internalized as something they can identify for themselves and over which they feel they have a greater degree of control such that the activation of the self–other representation can be nipped in the bud before it takes hold in the mind and potentially distorts the experience of current relationships.

Case example

Lara is a thirty-nine-year-old woman, referred because of recurrent depression and GAD. Things had become particularly difficult for her following the birth of her first child two years earlier. She described recurrent periods where she would feel "on a level" for a while but then would all of a sudden "hit a precipice" where she would become very agitated and low.

Lara recounted an uneventful early life, with no history of separation or trauma. She felt close to both of her parents until the age of around six when her younger brother was born. At that time, she had vivid recollections of her brother suddenly occupying all her mother's affections, and she and her sister being relegated to "second best." She remembered especially her mother as a critical and unsupportive person and her father as quiet and submissive. Her mother would often put her down about the way she looked, her exam results, and dress sense. She remembered that after completing family chores, her mother would always "inspect" what they had done, eventually redoing the chores again to her own satisfaction. Around the age of ten she found herself marginalized from all the other girls in her class after a rather nasty whispering campaign about her. This was deeply hurtful for her. She had always been angry that her mother did not show interest in her or support her in this situation.

Lara presented in the initial sessions as plainly dressed. She sat on the edge of the seat and nervously drank from a water bottle. She would always apologize at the beginning of sessions for either being too early or too late and she intimated early on that she was "relieved" that she wasn't seeing a female therapist. It became clear from her INs that she often felt judged and criticized and put down by so-called successful women and mothers—calling herself "a geek." This had become much worse since she had become a mum—at toddlers groups she felt preoccupied that she was failing in relation to other mothers, perceiving herself as having the worst-behaved child and being the one who coped the least well with the demands of motherhood. She would often withdraw in depression and anger, which would be sublimated and passively expressed.

The IPAF that was eventually agreed on focused on a recurrent sense of self as a "flawed woman" and a recurrent view of the other being "critical and superior" that triggered a conscious affect of anxiety and that appeared to defend against anger. Through the course of the middle phase, the interpersonal events of the week would invariably center around a female friend or acquaintance in particular by whom she had felt slighted or judged and this provided a helpful opportunity for exploring the IPAF. It was apparent that she needed to revisit this pattern repeatedly, in its different guises, and never appeared to find this unhelpfully repetitive.

Lara's repeated apologetic gestures towards her therapist were explored in the transference revealing a constant sense that the therapist would be thinking that she was "a geek" and "weird" and the fantasy that the therapist was a skilled parent, had a notably attractive partner, obedient children, and a happy marriage.

By the ending phase of the therapy Lara had made considerable progress. She acknowledged that it was difficult to end the therapy and fantasized that the therapist would be relieved to find another patient, revealing her fear that she would be replaced in the therapist's mind. This was productively explored in the transference.

Working in the transference

We will not say very much about this here since we devote a whole chapter to this later (see Chapter 8), but it is nevertheless important to note that the interpretation of the transference is a central technique in the middle phase because it helpfully roots the therapist in working on, and through, the patient's *current* relationships.

In the initial phase there is some discussion about past relationships as these inform the elaboration of the IPAF. However, in the middle phase sessions, this is less of a focus. It may, of course, be very pertinent to the IPAF for a patient to discuss past relationships. However, on the whole, during the middle phase, the therapist strives to prioritize working on *current* significant relationships that demonstrate the activation of the IPAF. The therapist thus focuses on helping the patient explore the vicissitudes of the therapeutic relationship because for the duration of the sixteen sessions it often becomes a significant relationship in the patient's life. The therapist will make use of the experience and observation of the patient's ways of relating within the session to inform the understanding of his internal world of relationships. Where appropriate the therapist draws attention to this to highlight the enactment of the IPAF in the session.

Working with defenses

An important aspect of working through the IPAF involves helping the patient to identify the often unconscious "investment" in maintaining a particular self–other representation. The patient may, for example, complain that he feels belittled by others whom he experiences as haughtily superior, and yet he repeatedly recruits into his world people who treat him in this way. This may be because one of the "pay-offs" is that this way he remains the victim of others' criticism and he can sidestep owning his own arrogance.

As we mentioned earlier, with some patients it is only in the middle phase that the therapist will share with them her understanding of the defenses they deploy and of the pay-offs afforded by the defensive configuration. In the middle phase a core strategy is therefore to help the patient to explore the defenses mobilized in relationships, including the unconscious strategies he uses to manage areas of difficulty in his relationships. The overall aim is to help the patient to reflect on behaviors and feelings that give rise to, perpetuate, or exacerbate the core interpersonal pattern identified by the IPAF.

Any behavior or feeling can be used defensively, that is, whatever allows for an alleviation of psychic pain belongs under the heading of defense. It is the psychic function of a behavior or feeling that determines whether it is being used defensively, for example, whether it protects self-esteem.

Defenses are often used to manage interpersonal anxiety generated, for instance, by a fear of being taken over or controlled by the other or of becoming too intimate. Such object-related defenses are, once again, varied. For example, some people may use distancing to protect themselves from intimacy; others may become obstinate as a way of controlling the object; and others still may become passive as a way of discharging hostility. There are also defenses that destroy or attack a mental process and leave the patient bereft of his own mental capacities (e.g. attacks on thinking as a defense against understanding something painful) and defenses that destroy a mental representation (e.g. splitting the representation of a significant other, reducing them to a part-object).

Defenses act as the gateway to change: flexible defenses that are open to challenge allow for a destabilization of the psychic status quo that maintains the problems. Rigid defenses, instituted to protect the individual from intolerable psychic pain, may prove harder to shift. A session-by-session assessment of defenses is critical for determining the patient's ability to respond to an interpretation. It is thus important to assess the balance between defense and motivation alongside the strength of the therapeutic alliance in every session.

If interpretation elicits more defensive behavior, this is suggestive of an entrenched defensive system that might well prove hard to shift in a brief intervention. If the interpretation of defense leads to regressive behavior on the part of the patient, this would suggest the possibility of defenses protecting the patient from a breakdown. For example, after the first session during which the therapist had made a trial interpretation, a patient reported going on a drinking binge that resulted in him losing consciousness. The urgent need in this patient to obliterate the session in his mind placed him at risk. In such cases it is advisable to proceed cautiously, to consider seriously the suitability for a more exploratory approach and, if continuing, this would be a strong indicator of the need to strengthen the supportive aspects of the approach until there is more evidence of ego strength.

The exploration of defenses is closely linked to the exploration of the patient's affect. Here we are primarily interested in helping the patient to become aware of several facets of his emotional life, namely (a) those affects that need to be kept in check by defenses, (b) those affects that function as defenses, that is, affects that protect the individual from feeling other emotional states, and (c) how particular affects are managed or discharged (e.g. through self-harm or substance abuse).

Working with defenses can be thought of as consisting of four interlinked strategies that build on each other: (a) the acceptance and validation of the need for defenses, (b) the exploration of the *how* of defenses (i.e., the patient's characteristic defensive strategies), (c) the exploration of the *why* of defenses (i.e., the function of defenses), and finally (d) the *costs* of defenses (see Figure 6.4) (Greenson, 1967).

Working through the defenses associated with the IPAF thus begins with an initial acceptance by the therapist of the patient's style of relating, that is, by communicating respect for the defensive needs that may underlie particular interpersonal styles. This can be facilitated through helping the patient to explore and become more aware of areas of conflict by drawing attention to feelings/states of mind that

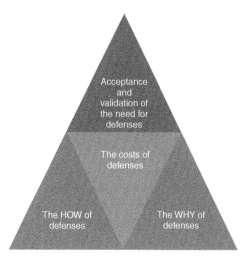

Figure 6.4 Strategies for exploring defenses.

seem unacceptable or uncomfortable without any pressure to change, at this stage.

It is in this context of acceptance that the therapist can then start to focus on helping the patient to understand *how* he protects himself from particular painful feelings/states of mind, for example, by empathically pointing out how he becomes confused or "unable to think."

Using the transference can help the patient to become more aware of how he manages problematic aspects of his relationships through an exploration of defenses as they arise in relation to the therapist and significant others. This will include helping the patient to manage the anxiety generated by the live exploration of defenses, which may feel very threatening to some.

Once the *how* of defenses has been explored, the therapist can move on to the *why* of defenses, that is, helping the patient understand why he needs to protect himself from the experience of particular feelings/ states of mind.

Finally, highlighting the *costs* of the defenses used by pointing out their impact on the patient's own capacities and on his relationships is a prerequisite for engaging the patient in relinquishing defenses: the costs need to outweigh the conscious and unconscious benefits if change is to occur.

Supporting attempts at new behavior in relationships

Insight into the unconscious relational patterns that inform the patient's behavior is a prerequisite for change, but it is often not sufficient in and of itself. Indeed many patients, though grateful for the clarity that the IPAF sheds on their difficulties, may yet turn round and say: "Yes, it all makes sense, but I still can't see what I can do to change."

Psychodynamic therapists do not all subscribe to the same view of what promotes psychic change. Some believe that change will be supported through assiduous attention to the transference dynamics; others maintain that this is achieved through the provision of a "new" relationship in the therapy; others still that it is through enhancing the patient's reflective capacity that change occurs and different techniques are thought to facilitate this. All of these processes may well be mutative, but in the absence of active support and focus on also trying out new ways of approaching the interpersonal scenarios that activate the IPAF, it may prove very hard for the patient, *in a brief period of time*, to leave the therapy with some confidence that he *can* actually respond differently in his current relationships.

Working in the transference provides a valuable opportunity for "practicing," as it were, two of the key "skills" that we hope to impart to the patient during a course of DIT, namely noticing the activation of a relational pattern and the associated affect, and using this enhanced self-reflective capacity to create the possibility for a different response. Practicing these skills in the transference is important, but the therapeutic relationship is often (though not always, of course) also experienced as a relatively safer place within which to take interpersonal risks. Consequently it may be more difficult for the patient to generalize this learning to other relationships.

Moreover, although with some patients the therapeutic relationship may very rapidly become the focus of their imaginative life and feelings, with others the transference is not always sufficiently emotionally live to provide adequate opportunities to work on these dynamics over sixteen sessions, and hence the patient's external relationships may carry greater affectivity and relevance and help to consolidate change. From the patient's point of view, exposure in the transference therefore needs to be reinforced with attempts at novel behavior in his current relationships outside of the therapy.

The exploration with the therapist of the success or failure of the patient's attempt at change offers yet more opportunity to understand the interpersonal and affective processes that inhibit change. Anticipating with the patient what may prove difficult is an integral part of the process of supporting change.

We are emphasizing that the therapist actively supports the patient to try out different ways of responding. The timing of this, however, will vary depending on the patient and how he is progressing during the middle phase. Absence altogether of any overt attempts at engaging the patient in trying out different ways of relating to others would nevertheless suggest that the therapist is not practicing DIT.

Chapter 7

Techniques

A key intervention in DIT, as we saw in Chapter 5, is to help the patient to stay focused on the agreed IPAF. All the techniques deployed in DIT support this core aim, that is, of helping the patient to better understand what is happening for him, in his mind, when things go wrong in his relationships. This will include, as we have seen, how the IPAF is enacted in the therapeutic relationship. To this end DIT draws on expressive/exploratory, supportive, mentalizing, and directive techniques, which we will now review.

Listening with an analytic ear

Before we can intervene we have to listen. Tuning into unconscious communication is not a passive process. It involves actively being with the patient, moment by moment, and tracking the changes in his states of mind, which indicate shifting identifications and projections. These changes are imperceptible to the untrained ear.

Listening to unconscious communication is demanding. It requires patience because unconscious meaning is seldom immediately obvious. Not only can an aspect of the environment, or its image, be used metaphorically, but also the people the patient refers to may represent— stand in for, as it were—other people. Sometimes they may represent the patient himself as a whole or as a part.

In the evolving conscious and unconscious dialogue between patient and therapist, the patient gives voice to complex schemata of self and other that indicate the activation contemporaneously, or in sequence, of different states of mind. For example, an experience of the self as a child raging at a punitive parent may give way to an experience of the self as a child yearning for an absent parent. Within the same session the patient may then oscillate between feeling the subject of angry impulses and, at other times, he may feel like the object of someone else's neglect. These shifts are seldom conveyed directly through language, but we can infer them from the stories patients recount and, importantly, *how* they recount them.

There are numerous vehicles for unconscious communication that are nonverbal, for example, posture, gesture, movement, facial expression, tone, syntax, rhythm of speech, pauses, and silences. Gestures, including bodily postures and movements, always accompany the speech process. The power of gestural messages rests precisely in the concealment that they afford and so become ideal vehicles for the communication of unconscious mental contents (Fonagy and Fonagy, 1995).

The patient's "ideolect" (Lear, 1993) endows the conscious narrative with unconscious resonances. Patients' preconscious attitudes are often expressed at the paralinguistic level preceding their emergence in the patients' verbal utterances. Meaning and unconscious fantasies may be expressed through the way the patient speaks rather than in what he says: a harsh tone, a soft, barely audible voice, or a fast-paced delivery can convey far more about the patient's psychic position at a given point in time than the words themselves.

The *how* of the patient's narrative also alerts us to the importance of its structure. The attachment research by Main and colleagues draws our attention to the meaning that is inherent in the organization of language itself. Main and Goldwyn (1998) make an explicit distinction between coherent and incoherent narratives. They distinguish between language that is collaborative and coherent and language that is incoherent, distorted, or vague. Incoherent narratives make it necessary for the listener to infer linkages of which the speaker may be unconscious so as to create organization and to deduce real or underlying meaning in the story that is being told. This distinction encourages us to listen closely to moment-to-moment changes in linguistic fluency and to shifts in voice, to lapses in meaning and coherence, and to the fragmentation of the narrative, all of which have been found in research studies to be indicators of attachment insecurity in adult speech (Main et al., 1985).

Listening to the structure of the patient's narrative sensitizes us to the quality of the patient's early experiences of attachment (Slade, 2000), and how this might be translated into the patient's current relationships. Secure or reflective patterns of language and thought indicate the presence of an internalized other who can contemplate or contain the breadth and complexity of the child's needs and feelings (Fonagy, 2001). In this sense, the breaks, incoherencies, and contradictions observed in the narratives of insecurely attached adults are said to imply a break in the caregiver's capacity to respond to the child's need for care and comfort.

Analytic listening, unlike ordinary listening, therefore takes place simultaneously on multiple levels and in reference to multiple contexts. This kind of layered listening acknowledges the complexity of the patient's communications and the hidden agendas. It not only underscores the central importance of the therapist's receptivity to the patient's conscious and unconscious communications, but also points to a key aspect of analytic listening, namely that it is impossible to listen without involving ourselves. This confronts us with a paradox:

> It is necessary for the analyst to feel close enough to the patient to feel able to empathise with the most intimate details of his emotional life: yet he must be able to become distant enough for dispassionate understanding. This is one of the most difficult requirements of psychoanalytic work—the alternation between the temporary and partial identification of empathy and the return to the distance position of the observer. (Greenson, 1967: 279)

Bollas (1996) approaches this dual demand on the therapist by distinguishing two types of listening, which he refers to respectively as the "maternal mode" and the "paternal mode." The maternal mode denotes a more receptive, "holding" therapeutic stance whereas the paternal mode reflects a more active and interpretative therapeutic stance. Bollas argues that both modes play complementary roles in the analytic process and this is certainly the case in DIT, which calls for different stances at different stages of the therapy, and sometimes within the same session. For example, if a patient is very distressed he may require us to operate in a more "maternal" mode than during times when he can withstand a more challenging exploration of the IPAF. Neither stance is better than the other; rather, they complement each other. This takes us back to the importance of the therapist's ability to implement DIT in a flexible way so as to respond to the patient's changing needs.

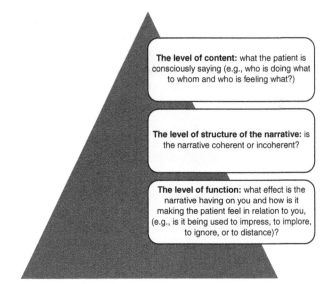

The level of content: what the patient is consciously saying (e.g., who is doing what to whom and who is feeling what?)

The level of structure of the narrative: is the narrative coherent or incoherent?

The level of function: what effect is the narrative having on you and how is it making the patient feel in relation to you, (e.g., is it being used to impress, to implore, to ignore, or to distance)?

Figure 7.1 Levels of listening.

Monitoring multiple levels of discourse simultaneously is essential. Communication, however, would fail if we did not take the first level of implication of what the patient says to us at face value. An over-emphasis on what the patient is not explicitly saying to the exclusion of what they *are* saying does not contribute to the development of a good therapeutic alliance. In DIT the therapist's interventions ideally convey an acknowledgement of both the manifest content of what the patient communicates and the possible latent content. Patients are less likely to feel misunderstood, bemused, or angered by our interpretation of unconscious meaning if we acknowledge first what they have actually said before making a link to its possible unconscious meaning (Figure 7.1).

Emergence versus structure in the sessions

A range of techniques support DIT's organizing principles and aims, namely to intervene so as to generate, clarify, and elaborate interpersonally relevant information and to encourage the patient's curiosity to reflect on what happens in his mind. All techniques "structure," to an extent, a session, in so far as whatever we do, or don't do, has a structuring impact on the therapeutic interaction. Obviously, some techniques impose far more structure than others.

One of the delicate balancing acts for the DIT therapist is that between allowing space, and hence silences, within which the unconscious aspects of the patient's experience can be elaborated, as we have been describing, and the necessary requirement to be more active and focused, which inevitably introduces a degree of structure into the sessions that may well, at first, feel rather alien. Listening to a DIT session nevertheless feels very different from listening to a CBT session because of the more emergent quality of the patient–therapist dialogue that is characteristic of DIT.

The more questions we ask, the more we structure the dialogue. Although clarificatory questions, as we shall shortly see, are encouraged in DIT, equally we are interested in what emerges more spontaneously in the patient's mind; and for this to happen we need to allow the patient some space. So let us be clear: there is room for silence in DIT.

At times silence indicates a quiet, reflective mood, which is beneficial or even necessary so as to allow for the emergence of latent affect. At other times it can be a sign of resistance or an attack. The pregnant pauses may also feel like a pressure to relieve the patient from his own introspection or the responsibility of thinking for himself. No matter how difficult silences may feel we must caution against premature impingement and pressurizing the patient to overcome them. We, too, of course, may use silence as a way of discharging our own hostility towards a patient. Therefore it is important to monitor our own silence and ensure it does not veer into withholding or neglect and perpetuate a misalliance.

Having said all this, given the time-limited nature of DIT, its focus and its aim to help the patient to effect some changes in his life, frequent, protracted silences would be very unusual in a prototypical DIT session.

Expressive/exploratory techniques

Once we have tuned into listening with an analytic ear, the therapist makes use of expressive/exploratory techniques to engage the patient in reflecting on what is being communicated. These techniques used in DIT will be familiar to all psychodynamically trained clinicians, namely confrontation, clarification, and interpretation. This technical constellation has a long history and can be traced back to Greenson's (1967) classic text on psychoanalytic technique. In our view it provides a helpful reminder to the therapist of a sequence of interventions, underlining that interpretation is a process (see the section below, Features of helpful interpretations)—that is, we gradually put in place the steps building up towards an interpretation. At its best this process means that the patient can be helped to arrive at his own interpretation.

Confrontation

The first stage in helping the patient to work through the IPAF is to create a shared "marker" of the issue that requires further clarification so as to gather the information we need to formulate an eventual interpretation. In other words, the therapist brings to the patient's attention the ostensible problem (e.g. lateness for sessions) to engage him in recognizing that there is something to be understood, that is, she confronts the patient with this "fact."

For example, one patient arrived very late for one of her sessions, which had followed a cancellation by the therapist the previous week. As she sat down, she looked very low and said she had been feeling more depressed than usual—a deterioration that was also reflected in her depression questionnaire scores. The therapist had a very clear idea in her mind about the lateness because it had followed her own cancellation and she thought this was of significance to this patient given the IPAF. She hypothesized that this patient might be sensitized to cancellations in a very particular way since the IPAF identified a self-representation as "insignificant" and an other-representation as "neglectful." Despite the therapist's conviction about the meaning of the lateness, in DIT she would be discouraged from jumping in with an interpretation without first ensuring that the patient recognizes that her lateness is a problem.

Let us now follow the progressive efforts the therapist made before sharing an interpretation. The therapist began by straightforwardly confronting the patient with the fact of her lateness. The deterioration in her symptomatic depression scores, along with her self-report of lowered mood at the start of the session, were also important signs and deserved acknowledgment:

> T: I can see from your scores and what you have said to me that you have been feeling more depressed than usual. And today you also arrived unusually very late—what do you make of this?
> P: I haven't been good at all . . . don't know why really . . . it goes in cycles . . . don't know about the lateness . . . I know you said it was important to have all the sessions and all that, but I just didn't get my act together this morning . . .

The therapist at this stage is factual, but immediately engages the patient in reflecting on the *meaning* behind her scores and her behavior (i.e., the lateness): "What do you make of this?" The patient does not elaborate at all in her response, but she nevertheless reveals that she knows getting to her sessions on time is important and that it is what the therapist has encouraged her to do. She does not dismiss the lateness as insignificant—she simply says she does "not know" about it. The therapist takes this as a cue for *clarifying* the interpersonal scenario that has arisen in the here-and-now.

Clarification

Clarificatory questions or statements allow the therapist to engage the patient in exploring the problem that is now openly acknowledged: "I have been arriving late and this is getting in the way of making use of the therapy." Clarificatory interventions serve to bring this problem into focus. They are apparently simple, yet underrated techniques.

Questions, traditionally, have been discouraged in psychodynamic practice, typically out of a concern that they introduce too much direction or they avoid the elaboration of painful affect. There is some truth in this, some of the time, with some patients. For example, asking questions may be used to fill in uncomfortable silences, but this is not an intrinsic quality of therapist-initiated questions. Some of the turning points in DIT are heralded not by the interpretation of transference, but by asking the kinds of questions that engage the patient in thinking deeply about what is happening in his mind, or that draw his attention to a detail that speaks volumes but that he had ignored.

An appropriately timed question that invites the patient to pause and reflect can be mutative and has the added advantage that it does not present the patient with the therapist's more fully formed formulation (in the form of an interpretation); rather it invites the patient to actively engage with his mind. This is why we encourage therapists to ask questions in order to clarify the patient's experience in his relationships and to help the patient to elaborate his mental states. Particular emphasis is placed on using clarificatory prompts to help the patient to reflect on unverbalized feelings. Here, as elsewhere in DIT, we make use of our own emotional reactions to the patient as a basis for facilitating this type of exploration.

Let us return to the patient who is very late for her session:

> T: I think it would be helpful to try to make some sense of what's been happening in your mind over the last two weeks because I am concerned that you are feeling worse. And although we don't yet know what made you late today, perhaps this is not irrelevant, and may help us to better understand how you have been feeling.
>
> P: I don't really know why I am late . . . I got up on time, and had set plenty of time aside to get here for 10 a.m. and then I ended up tidying up the house and by the time I looked at my watch I realized I was running fifteen minutes late. I don't know why I did that because then I felt anxious about being late.
>
> T: OK, so it sounds like you clearly had the session in mind when you got up this morning. And then something else started to happen in your mind . . . can you recall what went on? [silence]
>
> P: I was listening to the radio over breakfast and it was some discussion about soft sentencing for child abusers. Some woman was banging on about how the perpetrators are *victims* [the patient said this word in a dismissive way and carried on expressing her outrage at this, shaking her head] . . . I don't know what this has got to do with being late here though . . .
>
> T: You feel outraged and very angry with this woman because you felt she was ignoring the plight of the victims . . . [patient interrupts]
>
> P: Well, it's all very well being sympathetic to the abuser. I'm sure they've had a tough time and all that, but what about their victims—who's got *them* in mind?
>
> T: There is something in this radio interview that is so important to you and relevant to what we have been working on here: someone neglecting the needs of others who deserve and need care but who are somehow not kept in mind, who are insignificant . . .
>
> P: Yes, that really gets to me—there are so many invisible people in the world. Take the homeless on the streets . . . [patient continues in this gist]

In this example we can see how the therapist gradually draws in the patient to elaborate the events of the morning that preceded her late arrival for her session. The radio interview is recounted with very live affect and strikes the therapist as especially relevant. The therapist speculated that her cancellation of the patient's session had activated the patient's IPAF, casting the patient back into the familiar experience of feeling "insignificant" to the object and casting the therapist as the "neglectful other." In the event she was correct but the process of clarification was important not only because it substantiates the therapist's hypothesis through the narrative about the woman on the radio who neglects the invisible victims, but also because it engages the patient in a process of reflection that would be bypassed if the therapist just delivered her "correct" interpretation. Indeed, the patient arrives at the important realization that she reacts to situations where people are treated as "invisible" even though this important insight is immediately diluted by the patient's digression into a discussion about world poverty. This term "invisible" struck the therapist as even more emotionally accurate as the self-representation descriptor than "insignificant."

Clarificatory questions also provide an important corrective because it is all too easy for us to be seduced by the spoken word or by the assumption of shared meaning. Words carry with them a personal and uniquely individual meaning. In order to understand what our patients are trying to communicate, we need to check what they are intending. We can only do so by gently questioning something that appears to make sense, but may instead conceal a great deal that doesn't yet make sense.

Interpretation

Once the matter of the patient's lateness and its context has been sufficiently elaborated through clarificatory techniques, the therapist uses interpretation to address the dimension of the IPAF that is closest to the patient's current awareness and that has a bearing on the lateness. Where appropriate, the therapist makes a linking interpretation between the IPAF and the symptoms to help the patient to identify the relationship between symptoms and the activation of the IPAF. Given the brief nature of the intervention the focus of interpretation is primarily (but not exclusively) on pre-conscious material rather than more deeply unconscious or distal events.

Let us return to our working example:

> T: You used just now an important word: "invisible." And it made me think that perhaps it captures even more closely the position you often find

yourself in: that *you* become invisible to others, that your needs are not recognized and this makes you feel very angry and then you withdraw.

P: I had not really thought about that, but yes, invisible actually is what it feels like . . . invisible . . . with no voice . . . sometimes I feel like screaming but nothing comes out.

T: Yes, this does make sense because feeling you have no voice is part of the problem, which then makes it hard for you to tackle what is distressing you in a relationship. For example, here I have been wondering whether it has been hard for you to find a voice today to tell me how you really feel about me canceling your session a few weeks ago. You haven't directly mentioned this, but I think that when I canceled the session, this left you feeling that I was neglecting you, not "seeing" you and your needs. We know from the work we have been doing together here that when you feel "invisible" in this way this leads you to withdraw, which is perhaps why you were late today. I wonder if this is what may have led you to feel even more depressed over the last few weeks. Does this make any sense to you?

An interpretation is a *hypothesis*. It invites the patient to comment on it, if he wishes to, or to ignore it. This is why an interpretation is ideally couched as a tentative statement, question, or formulation that conveys to the patient, "This might be one way of understanding what you are saying. What do you think?" An interpretation is not a statement of truth where we tell the patient what he is *really* thinking even if he does not yet know it; rather, it is an invitation to consider another perspective which may, or may not, fit.

Interpretations in DIT can focus on a wide range of thoughts, feelings, or behavior:

+ They can draw attention to contradictory "versions" of people, including the therapist, and the anxieties that lie behind the construction of such contradictory representations.

+ They can address specific defensive maneuvers that compromise the patient's self-awareness and connection to the therapist in the session, that is, transference interpretations.

+ They can be directed at the patient's self and other representations, helping him to explore positive and negative attributes.

+ They can center on the identification of patterns in the patient's actions, thoughts, and feelings, especially as they relate to the IPAF.

It is important to remember that the process of interpretation aims not only to capture the patient's conscious and unconscious experience,

Box 7.1 Characteristics of helpful questions

Helpful questions:

♦ Are relevant to the agreed IPAF and support its elaboration

♦ Encourage reflection on and elaboration of mental states, underlying interpersonal experiences and the patient's moods, including the active consideration of alternative assumptions and perspectives

♦ Encourage the patient to consider alternative ways of behaving in response to his interpersonal difficulties

but also to introduce a new perspective on his experience by sharing the therapist's view of things. This is best achieved in an open-minded and questioning rather than dogmatic way, modeling exploration, and adding meaning in a flexible way, thus stimulating the patient's confidence in, and use of, his own self-reflective capacities (Box 7.1).

Finally, when interpreting we always need to keep in mind that even though an interpretation is a hypothesis, it can nevertheless be experienced by the patient as an action, that is, as the therapist *doing* something to the patient. For example, an interpretation of the unconscious motivation that may lie behind the patient's investment in the IPAF could be experienced as the therapist making a critical comment. Knowing when and what to interpret thus relies on our ongoing assessment of the patient's shifting states of mind, within a given session, and over time, which will determine how he hears an interpretation. It also requires that we are attuned to the patient's experience of an interpretation and can respond to this with empathy and curiosity.

Features of helpful interpretations

A good interpretation is simple, to the point, and transparent. By "transparent" we mean that the interpretation shows the patient how we have arrived at our particular understanding. This is especially important in the early stages of DIT when the patient might be unaccustomed to working with the unconscious, and may therefore experience an interpretation as "plucked out of the blue" unless it is grounded in the context of what he has been talking about in the session.

The therapist works collaboratively with the patient to facilitate his active involvement in the process of self-understanding. Questions and observations that stimulate the patient's own self-reflective process are prioritized over interpretations of deep unconscious content that may contribute to the patient's experience of being the passive recipient of the therapist's understanding.

A core aim of interpretation in DIT is to stimulate the generation of multiple perspectives on the patient's predicament. The therapist takes the many opportunities provided by the patient's description of real-life interpersonal incidents to help the patient to exercise flexible understanding of the possible feelings and thoughts (of the different individuals involved), getting the patient to elaborate different internal scenarios perhaps underlying these incidents, questioning habitual assumptions.

In considering the task of interpretation we thus need to think about two aspects: the *process* of interpreting and the *content* of interpretations. As we have already suggested, interpretation in DIT is best seen as a process (i.e., based on a series of interventions over time, rather than on a single comment). The therapist draws on the use of clarification and confrontation to gradually bring feelings, fantasies, and behaviors to the patient's attention and as the basis for eventually making an interpretation (Box 7.2). This involves a number of related strategies:

- Helping the patient to explore and become more aware of painful conflicts by pointing out unacceptable or uncomfortable feelings that are otherwise managed by being kept out of the patient's conscious awareness.

- Drawing the patient's attention to communication that is unclear, vague, puzzling, or contradictory with the aim of encouraging the patient to elaborate on these elements.

- Helping the patient become aware of incongruent elements in his communication by pointing out and giving meaning to discrepancies and incongruities in what is being communicated through different "channels" (e.g. a contrast between verbal and nonverbal communication).

Box 7.2 Characteristics of helpful interpretations

- *Clear* (i.e., succinct enough for the patient to be able to take in what is being said)
- *Appropriately timed* (a) in relation to an assessment of what the patient can bear to think about at any given point, and (b) relative to the amount of time left in a session (i.e., not introducing new topics that may be unsettling to the patient too close to the end of a session)
- *Of appropriate depth* (i.e., moving gradually from preconscious content to more unconscious content)
- *Pertinent* to the affective-interpersonal focus of the session
- Framed in a *tentative way* such that the patient is invited to discuss rather than necessarily agree with the therapist's view

- Identifying and pointing out to the patient unverbalized affect when it is manifested in the session.

Focusing on affect

The IPAF contains an important affective dimension and throughout DIT we are closely attentive to the patient's emotional experience. We listen not only to the affect present in the content of what the patient says, but also to the affect that is communicated through the process of the joint interaction in the room.

Our aim is to facilitate the expression of unexpressed or unconscious feelings by communicating to the patient that his feelings can be tolerated and thought about by us (i.e., through the therapist's understanding, empathic stance) and by responding to the patient's nonverbal cues and linking these to unexpressed or unconscious feelings.

The therapist enquires into the subjective meaning of the patient's use of particular words, dreams, fantasies, or nonverbal behaviors to help to focus the exploration on the patient's affective experience, drawing attention to the internal and interpersonal obstacles to the awareness, and expression, of particular feelings (especially in the context of the relationship with the therapist).

Many of our interventions throughout DIT essentially aim to help the patient to:

- identify what he feels, encouraging the patient to stay with a current feeling as it emerges in the session
- communicate what he feels more effectively
- build greater facility in connecting his feelings, thoughts, and actions, and how these relate to others' internal states and behavior.

The affective dimension of the IPAF is integral to the working through of the IPAF. The therapist thus strives to help the patient to identify the way in which his feelings are guided by the particular self and other representation that is activated in a given relationship. The patient's conscious affect, though important given that this is what the patient feels troubled by, as we have observed before (see Chapter 5), may yet conceal latent affect that may be even more disturbing to the patient.

Supportive techniques

No therapy can occur without some supportive techniques. Support and empathy are necessary components of all therapies. Because DIT is brief, is used with patients with moderately severe problems, and aims to engage the patient very quickly, supportive interventions are an integral part of the approach. In practice this means that it is important to start with a basic supportive stance and to work towards making more demands on the patient's capacity for self-reflection over time. The therapeutic skills of reflective listening and accurate empathy are a fundamental aspect of DIT. This does not mean that we agree with everything the patient says. Confrontation or challenge is an equally important aspect of DIT.

Because DIT is used with patients whose depression and/or anxiety may be comorbid with Axis II disorders, the therapist needs to titrate the level of supportive interventions offered to a given patient. The less impaired patient, with a higher level of premorbid interpersonal functioning, is more likely to make greater use of expressive/exploratory techniques without requiring more supportive interventions to bolster defenses and support his day-to-day functioning. The ability to apply the model flexibly and to balance supportive and expressive techniques is therefore essential.

Mentalizing interventions

Mentalization-focused interventions within DIT aim to support a therapeutic process in which the mind of the patient is the focus of the treatment. As we have been emphasizing, the objective is for the patient to find out more about *how* (not just what) he thinks and feels about himself and others, how that dictates his responses, and how "errors" in understanding himself and others lead to (unhelpful) actions in an attempt to retain stability and to make sense of incomprehensible feelings.

How to identify failures of mentalizing

The process of addressing mentalization problems begins with the therapist identifying a break in mentalizing. But how does a therapist know when such a break has occurred? This obviously takes some practice and experience but being familiar with the smooth coherent discourse of a mentalizing narrative is a helpful start. Box 7.3 displays some of the features of good mentalizing. It is helpful to note that many of the features, such as acknowledgment of the inherent opaqueness of what someone else thinks or feels, is something that we normally take for granted in daily conversations—not just in therapeutic contexts.

In the context of psychotherapy we typically encounter at least two common types of nonmentalizing discourse. These are rooted in two different modes of experiencing subjectivity that emerge in place of mentalizing. The most common is what we refer to as *psychic equivalence*. In theoretical terms this refers to patients treating mental reality as if it was identical to outer reality. In psychic equivalence what is experienced as mental or internal acquires the potency of phenomena happening in the physical world. There is a rigid mode of thinking in which the patient has the conviction of privileged access to the true state of affairs. Interpersonally this mode of thinking inevitably leads to significant problems with conflict because the patient

Box 7.3 What does good mentalizing look like in relation to other people's thoughts and feelings?

- Acknowledgement of opaqueness
- Absence of paranoia
- Contemplation and reflection
- Perspective taking
- Genuine interest
- Openness to discovery
- Understanding and forgiveness of others
- Predictability
- Perception of own mental functioning
- Appreciation of changeability
- Developmental perspective
- Realistic skepticism
- Acknowledgment of preconscious function
- Awareness of impact of affect
- Self-presentation, e.g. autobiographical continuity
- General values and attitudes, e.g. tentativeness and moderation

cannot accept the validity of alternative perspectives ("I know exactly what the solution is and no one can tell me otherwise"). Finding "fault" in the other replaces self-reflection. Indeed, perhaps most characteristic of psychic equivalence is the attitude of certainty the patient has about the content of the other's mind. While his accounts of his own mental states are barren, he expresses a great deal of certainty about the thoughts or feelings of others. The accounts may be simplistic and dominated by description of acts that masquerade as causation. Such certainty often comes at a price. For example, self-related negative cognitions in psychic equivalence feel very real indeed and feelings of badness are experienced with unbearable intensity.

In psychic equivalence mental states are rarely part of the explanation of actions. The narrative consists of concrete descriptions of events without extensive consideration of their psychological motives. The patient appears not to have an appreciation of the feelings of self or others or of the relationships between thoughts, feelings, and actions. There is a general lack of attention to the thoughts, feelings, and wishes of others. When eliciting INs, in the absence of an acknowledgment of the thoughts and feelings of those whose actions are being described, the patient may relate excessive detail about the events to the exclusion of the other's psychological motivations. In explanations the patient is likely to focus excessively on external/social factors, such as the motives of institutions (the school, the council, the neighbors). Even when mental states are noted the patient typically concentrates on what are observable or undifferentiated character descriptions (e.g. tired, lazy, clever, self-destructive, depressed, has a short fuse). Another indicator of this type of concrete mentalizing rooted in psychic equivalence is a preoccupation with social concerns that do not require consideration of mental states, for example, a concern with rules, responsibilities, "shoulds," and "should nots."

Another type of nonmentalizing is the manifestations of the *pretend mode* of subjectivity. In a sense this complements psychic equivalence where ideas are too real—in pretend mode they do *not* feel real. In this mode of subjectivity the patient's ideas do not bridge inner experience with outer reality, leaving his mental world partially decoupled from external reality. This means that he can talk about thoughts and feelings more freely than is usual. More or less anything can be said without it carrying true meaning or containing genuine appropriate affect. The term *pseudo-mentalizing* has been used to describe this type of therapeutic discourse: it looks like mentalizing but is evidently missing one or more essential features of genuine mentalizing. In its most extreme manifestation, the subjective experience is likely to be one of emptiness and general meaninglessness. The lack of reality associated with internal experience permits unrealistic and unwarranted leaps of speculation about the mental states of others. In therapy endless inconsequential talk of thoughts and feelings might occur. Perhaps the clearest indicator that this mode is operative is that feelings do not accompany thoughts in the way we might expect, and understanding of the reasons for actions lacks conviction in relation to both one's own and others' actions.

The pretend mode can manifest in narratives as *intrusive mentalizing* when the patient makes wild assumptions about the mental states of others, failing to respect the inherent opacity of the mental states of others. In some instances the thoughts and feelings talked about may be somewhat plausible and even roughly accurate, but the therapist notices that they are assumed without the appropriate qualification ("I can't be certain, but it strikes me that . . .").

Nonmentalizing is more obvious when the patient makes lots of effort to understand actions in mental state terms, and may even appear to have a kind of preoccupation with mental state explanations, but these are somehow off the mark. The patient is not motivated to check the accuracy of his assumptions about the states of mind that provide the foci for his interests. We have elsewhere termed this uninquisitive, yet prolific form of contemplating mental states in pretend mode *hypermentalization*. In some individuals pretend mode manifests in *destructively inaccurate* mentalizing, which denies the objective reality. Here the patient attempts to deny aspects of objective reality, for example, in a self-serving manner. For example, the patient may "explain" other people's negative reactions to his anger by attributing highly psychologically implausible mental states (e.g. "My boss is simply envious of my talents").

How to use mentalizing interventions

It is not the content but the process of understanding, feeling, and experiencing that is at the heart of this component of the intervention. From this perspective therefore it is not for the therapist to "tell" the patient about how he feels, what he thinks, how he should behave, what the underlying reasons are, conscious or unconscious, for his difficulties. We believe that any therapy approach which moves towards "knowing" how a patient "is," how he should behave and think, and "why he is like he is" carries the risk of being harmful for some individuals.

The mentalizing component of DIT underlines the therapist's inquisitive or "not-knowing" stance. It underscores an attitude of curiosity and open enquiry. It is also an attempt to capture a sense that mental states are opaque and that the therapist can have no more idea of what is in the patient's mind than the patient himself. But when we say that the therapist adopts a "not-knowing" stance this is not synonymous with having no knowledge. Indeed formulating the IPAF represents the therapist's understanding—albeit tentative—of what is troubling the patient.

When the therapist shares the IPAF or an interpretation, and this may involve taking a different perspective to the patient, this should be verbalized and explored in relation to the patient's alternative perspective, without making assumptions about whose viewpoint has greater validity. The task is to determine the feelings and thoughts that have led to alternative viewpoints and to consider each perspective in relation to the other, accepting that diverse outlooks are possible, sometimes inevitable.

The focus of mentalizing interventions is on affect. Such interventions are simple, always focusing on mind rather than behavior and as much as possible on current (in session) affect and experience. At her best the therapist provides a mentalizing model, required to own up to her own antimentalizing errors, which are treated as opportunities to learn more about feelings and experiences (e.g. "How was it that I did that at that time?"). When misunderstandings occur, for example, the therapist articulates what has happened in order to demonstrate that she is continually reflecting on what goes on in her mind.

The principal aims are always the same: to be aware of the loss of mentalizing, particularly when the patient is emotionally aroused, for example while talking about an intensely conflictual attachment relationship, and then to work to reinstate mentalizing (see Box 7.4). This is achieved by "rewinding," going back with the patient to the point in the narrative where mentalizing was lost. The temptation is to try to help the patient to "understand" nonmentalizing content: for example, his belief, based on a glance, that a friend hates him. The impression that a friend, who has been loyal and supportive, suddenly turned against him is nonmentalizing content and exploring it usually gets the therapeutic couple into a pretend mentalization process where the patient is creating mental contents that he does not truly believe in. In such instances it is often more productive to take the patient back to the moments before he had this feeling. For example, the patient may

Box 7.4 Steps in making an intervention

- Identify a break in mentalizing
- Rewind to a moment before the break in subjective continuity
- Explore the current emotional context in session by identifying the momentary affective state between patient and therapist
- Explicitly identify and own up to the therapist's contribution to the break in mentalizing
- Seek to understand the mental states implicit in the current state of the patient–therapist relationship (mentalize the transference)

remember thinking that he felt frustrated by the friend's anxiousness to please or was angry with some minor infraction of the friendship. Contextualizing the experience this way, and linking it to genuine mentalization, makes it far more likely that a meaningful understanding of the experience will emerge.

The therapeutic aim in such situations is to help the patient to stabilize mentalizing in the context of attachment relationships. By painstakingly working through the example above, the patient's capacity to understand how his mind works, to see how he can simply switch off thinking and start attending to clues of limited relevance and significance, which in turn can so profoundly disturb his experience in relationships, is of great generic value. It can be "marked as important" (usually by agreeing a shared memory handle for the experience—e.g. "that irritation thing") and used later in the same session or in later sessions as something to go back to. In general the therapist aims to help the patient to find such clues or signals to mentalization failure that might alert the patient that feelings and thoughts that follow such signals may be the consequences of poorly mentalized thinking on their part.

Of course mentalizing others can be helpful too. Identifying non-mentalizing thinking that explains others' actions often meets with far less resistance in the patient than applying this in relation to himself. The therapist might therefore choose strategically to formulate with the patient an example of failed mentalizing by someone other than the patient (usually an attachment figure) and only slowly encourage the patient to see this as something that might often happen in him too.

The mentalizing therapeutic stance includes: (a) humility deriving from a sense of "not-knowing;" (b) whenever possible taking time to identify difference in perspectives; (c) legitimizing and accepting different perspectives; (d) active questioning of the patient in relation to their experience—less demanding explanations ("why questions") than detailed descriptions of experience ("what questions"); and (e) eschewing the need to understand (particularly feeling an obligation to understand the non-understandable).

It should above all be remembered that in the course of a treatment there is a high likelihood of the therapist losing her capacity to mentalize in the face of a nonmentalizing patient. This may lead to an enactment. This is an acceptable concomitant of therapeutic alliance, something that simply has to be acknowledged and reflected upon. As with other instances of breaks in mentalizing the incident requires that the process is rewound and the incident explored (see also Chapter 9).

Communication analysis

This represents yet another intervention, which is not specific to DIT, since it is also used in IPT (and other approaches). We use it specifically in DIT because it supports our focus on enhancing mentalizing. Through communication analysis the patient is helped to reflect on his communication with others in order to identify ways in which he expresses (or denies) strong affects and to identify alternative strategies for managing interpersonal conflicts.

Communication analysis is especially helpful when the patient reports a difficult interpersonal exchange. It is a simple, but powerful technique that involves the therapist listening to a particular IN and then inviting the patient to pause and reflect on it in great detail. The emphasis here is on the movie-script level of detail that is gathered (e.g. "So when you said that, what did you feel? Do you think you conveyed to him how angry you felt? When he responded by walking off, what went through your mind?" etc.). Through the questions we ask, the interpersonal exchange is magnified in as live a manner as possible, with particular attention to the patient's affective experience and his mental states. Identifying unhelpful communication patterns often involves listening for the assumptions that the patient makes about another person's thoughts or feelings and what he feels about himself as he relates to the other person. The overall aim is to help the patient to communicate more effectively.

Directive interventions

Once the link to the IPAF has been established, we can use more directive interventions to support the translation of the patient's understanding of the IPAF into change in his current relationships. As we have noted before, from the outset, the therapist enlists the patient as a collaborative participant in the process, engaging him in actively working on his more acute problems. Such an endeavor, in the context of a time limit, requires the judicious use of more directive interventions.

The most "directive" intervention in DIT is the focus on the IPAF, which will require tracking the focus and actively redirecting the patient to it where necessary. But the therapist's greater activity also includes interventions such as the judicious use of psycho-education or actively helping the patient to solve interpersonal dilemmas. These kinds of more active interventions may well be less familiar to psychodynamic colleagues trained in long-term work, since they are generally proscribed in the context of such work. In DIT, however, interventions such as active encouragement to try out different ways of approaching a conflict with another person are considered to have a subtle structuring impact on the patient's perspective on his experience.

Let us look more closely at some of these more directive interventions and what they are *not*, since direct advice and suggestions are discouraged (although the therapist might exceptionally do so; for example, if a patient has been having suicidal thoughts, the therapist might make a plan with the patient about how to manage these if they happen outside the session).

Unlike CBT, where the patient may be asked to carry out specific homework tasks or keep diaries that are then reviewed in the next session, in DIT the therapist employs *nonspecific directives*. This is because, although homework can be very helpful, it does make particular demands on the patient, particularly if the patient is cognitively affected by depression. DIT does not make such demands on the patient.

Nonspecific directives allow the therapist to signal that action is needed and engage the patient in reflecting on what may stand in the way of progress. After having explored a problematic interpersonal scenario with a patient (say a difficult exchange with a partner, during which the patient felt he could not express what he was feeling), the therapist might, for example, say:

> You feel very stuck and you are clearly telling me this is causing you a lot of distress. The more you avoid talking with your partner about what's on your mind, the more you withdraw into yourself and then the more depressed you seem to feel. If you could replay this exchange what do you think you might do differently?

The therapist would then closely track what the patient might wish he could do differently and help him to identify the interpersonal "steps" that are required. Close attention is paid to the areas of vulnerability linked to the IPAF that stand in the way of change. Once this is clarified the therapist would straightforwardly ask the patient what he imagines might happen if he did try to put into practice a different way of engaging with his partner so as to anticipate some of the obstacles the patient might encounter.

Sometimes the patient will spontaneously report a scenario where he has tried out a different way of relating. It can be very helpful to extrapolate from a situation where the patient has found a constructive and novel solution, articulating the significance of this, so as to support some generalization of a more constructive way of managing relationships. But, of course, things do also go wrong and the therapist needs to be alert to this possibility and receptive to the patient's negative feelings about the therapy and the therapist when this happens.

Psycho-education is used very sparingly, but it can be helpful for some patients, especially in the initial phase, to orient them to the DIT's relational frame of reference and its focus on mental states. In other words, we don't educate the patient about his symptoms per se, but about a way of understanding his symptoms. For example, we might say to a patient who gets easily angry but who is unconvinced by the therapist's focus on his mind:

> I can appreciate that it might well be difficult at this stage to see how this might help, but what goes on in our minds—what we feel, think, imagine to be happening—all this actually informs how we relate to others, what we expect from them, and what we imagine they expect from us. So if we can get a better picture of what is going on in your mind when you lose your temper, for example, this might actually help you to not be pulled in that direction all the time, which is so distressing to you.

The use of directive techniques in DIT is always framed in the context of a good understanding of the meaning that the therapist's more directive stance may acquire for the patient in light of the IPAF. For example, an anxious patient for whom separation is felt to be terrifying may well be very compliant with the therapist's direction because noncompliance is felt to pose a threat to the relationship. Yet, in spite of the therapist's support and encouragement, little change occurs for this patient. In such an instance, the DIT therapist would be very attuned to the unconscious meaning that may be latent in the patient's wish to please the therapist and would actively take this up with the patient, linking it to the identified IPAF and the lack of progress in the therapy.

Chapter 8

Working in the Transference

Working in the transference is one of the cornerstones of psycho-dynamic technique and its interpretation is held by many to be the royal road to psychic change. As we saw in the previous chapter, a range of techniques is deployed in DIT but we consider that working in the transference is a fundamental intervention that facilitates the exploration of the IPAF. In DIT the therapist makes *systematic use of the transference*, that is, she monitors her experience of the transference and of her own countertransference in order to inform her understanding of the patient's state of mind and hence how to intervene. In practice this may entail *not* making a verbal interpretation. In our view, we should always "use" the transference as a compass to orient us in relation to the unfolding of the therapeutic process (Lemma, in press), but we need to carefully consider how its interpretation furthers the therapeutic aims at any given point in time and whether the patient can tolerate it. In this chapter we therefore outline how to formulate a transference interpretation and the rationale for doing so within DIT.

Using the transference to explore the IPAF

As deployed in DIT, a transference interpretation is an intervention that uses the here and now of the therapeutic interaction to bring to the patient's attention the activation in his mind of a specific representation of self in relation to an other, that is, the IPAF.

The transference can take many forms, for example, positive, idealized, negative, or sexualized. A transference interpretation makes explicit reference to the patient–therapist relationship and its particular quality at a given point in time. Working in the transference relies primarily on interpreting the *current* relationship between therapist and patient (i.e., as opposed to interpreting the childhood origins of the patient's current interpersonal patterns). In DIT we share this here-and-now focus, but we also make links and draw parallels between the patient's subjective experience with the therapist and that with current others outside the therapy and (and vice versa) to illustrate the relevance of the IPAF across different interpersonal contexts and temporal dimensions.

Whilst some patients become very quickly and consciously preoccupied in their own minds with the therapist, others do not and may find links to the therapeutic relationship irrelevant or even odd. Others may be quite consciously preoccupied with the therapist, but they do not find it easy to report on the therapeutic relationship. In order to support the elaboration of the IPAF the therapist actively encourages the patient to discuss and explore his perceptions of, and feelings about, her and how he thinks the therapist may feel or think about him. Working in the transference thus rests on our receptivity to the patient's view of us—however distorted this may be—so as to allow a particular experience of the patient's self in relationship to us to emerge in the session. This requires an ability to recognize the patient's need to "test" the relationship with us in the transference and to communicate this understanding to the patient who may be worried, for example, about our anticipated rejection.

There are a number of ways in which a transference interpretation can support the exploration and working through of the IPAF:

- Transference dynamics are live and more immediate, and hence more verifiable in the here and now than the patient's report of past experiences or relationships outside of the therapy. What the patient tells us has happened to him is subject to the distortions of memory. So, whilst this is a valuable source of information about what troubles the patient and how he manages his life, the information is inevitably once removed. By contrast, the relationship that develops with the therapist provides a more immediate experience of some of the interpersonal dynamics that occur outside the therapeutic relationship. It allows the therapist to make these conflicts explicit to the patient as they are happening in the room, thus providing raw material to reflect on with the patient.

- Some patients are very adept at telling stories, but they struggle with expressing affect. The transference interpretation allows the therapist to make use of the emotional immediacy of the therapeutic relationship to counter intellectual resistances. The immediacy of the interventions based on this more direct source of information can have a very profound, and often moving, effect on the patient.

◆ The transference interpretation facilitates an increase in interpersonal intimacy by allowing the therapist to demonstrate attunement to the patient's current experience. A well-timed and accurate transference interpretation is perhaps one of the most powerful expressions of the therapist's empathy, as it shows the patient that he has been heard at various levels, not only in terms of what once happened, but also in terms of what *is* happening. For those patients who have not had the experience of being with another person who reflects back to them what is only indirectly implied in their communications, a transference interpretation can be experienced as containing and transformative.

◆ The transference interpretation allows the therapist to address the patient's defenses against intimacy as they emerge in the therapeutic relationship and so contributes to a strengthening of the alliance. We all recognize that patients turn up for their sessions but this does not necessarily mean that they want to be there. The transference interpretation squarely focuses on the reasons why the patient may want to avoid the therapeutic relationship by trying to reflect on the anxieties it generates. At its best, this kind of interpretation helps the patient to move on from a resistance.

◆ Through a transference interpretation the therapist models a way of handling negative perceptions and interpersonal conflict. Many transference interpretations highlight the patient's negative perception and experience of the therapist. In making an interpretation that acknowledges these the therapist implicitly conveys to the patient that it is possible to reflect on such feelings without catastrophic consequences.

◆ Transference interpretations enhance the patient's capacity to recognize and think about his states of mind. Because they usually pull together strong but confusing feelings, and unconscious, distorted thoughts and behavior, the patient is helped to see the relevance and helpfulness of taking a new perspective, and understanding what is happening between him and an important other person.

For all the reasons just listed, a transference interpretation is a powerful intervention. This is why it is also important to evaluate its impact. As with any intervention we make it is essential to note and respond to the emotional impact of transference interpretations on the patient so that their use is "titrated" in a manner that reflects the patient's capacity to receive them. In a more general sense we work to understand and help the patient to manage the emotional impact on him of the transference relationship, where appropriate, because an increase in the patient's positive or negative feelings towards us may be experienced as confusing or frightening for the patient. To this end it is helpful to consider:

◆ The patient's conscious and unconscious response to the interpretation (e.g. what associations/understandings follow an interpretation).

◆ The therapist's evaluation of the quality of the working alliance following an interpretation (i.e., a strengthening or weakening of the alliance).

◆ The patient's level of distress following an interpretation (however "right" our interpretation, if the patient feels too persecuted by it, it is of no use to him).

Formulating a transference interpretation

Let's now look more closely at the components of a transference interpretation. For an interpretation to be useful to the patient, as we suggested in Chapter 7, it needs to make some sense rather than being experienced as coming out of the blue, apparently unconnected to what the patient has been saying. It is therefore helpful to start from the patient's conscious experience of what is transpiring between him and the therapist. In other words, such interpretations begin by *describing* the patient's experience, as in the following example of work with a patient whose IPAF identified a self-representation as "unlovable" and another representation as "cruel," with rage as the linking affect. Early on in this patient's thirteenth session, the therapist reminded her that they were now approaching the ending. The therapist had been mindful of this patient's difficulty with endings throughout the therapy, but even so, this patient responded to this reminder in a striking manner:

T: We have three more sessions left after today . . .

P: [The patient interrupts, stiffens in her posture, and looks taken aback] What do you mean?

T: You seem to be taken aback by my reference to the end of our work together as if I have just broken the news to you for the first time. [Silence]

P: [Dismissively] You must have mentioned it . . . but I have had more worrying things on my mind . . . I probably didn't take it in. It doesn't matter . . .

[At this stage the therapist has only responded to the patient's manifest communication. She then tries to engage the patient in clarifying and exploring the feelings that have been evoked in order to elaborate the experience:]

T: I have the strong feeling that it does actually matter to you even though I can see that it might feel easier to just ignore what you really feel about this . . .

P: What's the point of talking about it . . . it won't change the facts . . . it's not like you will offer me any more sessions . . . anyway it's fine . . .

T: We are on familiar territory here: you feel upset and you push me away because you anticipate that I'm not interested in your experience . . . [Silence]

P: I need to detach, otherwise it's too painful . . .

[Long silence and then patient becomes tearful]

T: Something does feel very painful . . .

P: I hate saying goodbye . . . my life has been littered with goodbyes or people turning their backs on me. I can't face another one here. I'd rather just get up and leave now—have done with it.

T: I can understand why that might seem like the least painful solution, right now. And it would also be you turning your back on me rather than me doing this cruel thing to you which, I think, is how it felt at the beginning of the session when I reminded you of the three sessions we have left . . .

P: [The patient sounds very brittle and angry] What is it to you anyway? You're a therapist and it's your job—nothing wrong with that, but at the end of the day it's just another ending for your notes. You won't even remember my name in a few weeks' time . . .

At this point the therapist has elicited enough information to make a link to the IPAF, that is, she can abstract the relational pattern that has been activated in the patient's mind by the ending of the therapy and its interpersonal implications:

> T: There seems to be room for only one script here: I'm a ruthless therapist who won't even remember your name and I'm abandoning you. You now feel like "just another patient," someone I can easily disregard, not someone I have grown to know well over the last few months and whose feelings about the ending are very important. But if we get stuck in this particular conversation we can't think together about how the ending feels for you and this only makes you feel more alone and abandoned by me.

How we share with the patient our understanding of the transference deserves some consideration. Of course we each have our own particular therapeutic style that influences how we present our interpretations to the patient and there is no "right" way of doing it since every patient is different and, to an extent, we always adapt our style accordingly. We have found that with some patients—especially those who are not acculturated to a psychological approach to their problems—it is helpful to present the transference dynamic as a kind of "internal conversation." For example, say we formulate that at a given point in a session the patient feels criticized by us and that his way of managing this is to become contemptuous of our interventions. In this scenario we might share our formulation in the following way:

> I think that when you experience me as critical in your mind you are no longer talking with someone who is on your side, but with someone who is attacking you. The only way you feel you can then protect yourself is by putting me down as if you are saying to me, "I don't need you any more. What you have to offer me is worthless."

If the patient finds this way of thinking congenial, the work of therapy can then be framed as aiming to help him to have different kinds of "internal" conversations which, in turn, can expand the range of the actual conversations he can allow in his external relationships.

Criteria for interpreting the transference in DIT

As we mentioned earlier, DIT makes active use of the here-and-now therapeutic interaction. However, this should not be taken to mean that all that is discussed is what transpires between therapist and patient—this would not be DIT as transference interpretations are

Box 8.1 Criteria for interpreting the transference in DIT

- When it enhances the exploration of the IPAF
- When making a link between the transference and an external relationship adds immediacy and validity to the work
- When the patient finds it difficult to report INs (or is very isolated) and hence what transpires between the patient and therapist is the most "live" material available to work with
- When the therapist considers that the IN reported by the patient is being used to create emotional distance from the IPAF and a transference interpretation about what is going on in the here and now serves to refocus the patient
- When there is a resistance to the work of therapy

used in a more circumscribed manner than in longer-term psychodynamic therapies.

Moreover, the aim of a transference interpretation in DIT is not only, or even primarily, to arrive at an insight; the equally important goal is to engage the patient in the process of making sense of how his mind works. Using what happens in the transference often provides the most immediate way of doing this, but there may also be other interpersonal experiences outside of the therapy that carry a strong affective charge and that could be equally useful to this end.

There are several cues for interpreting the transference in DIT (see Box 8.1):

1. The main rationale for interpreting the transference in DIT is *to enhance the exploration of the IPAF.* This means that the therapist is monitoring the extent to which the INs the patient brings carry sufficient emotional immediacy to support the exploration of the IPAF or whether the IPAF can be more clearly discerned within the context of the therapeutic dyad and with greater immediacy.

2. There may be occasions when the therapist deems that making a link between the transference and an external relationship

adds immediacy and validity to the work, or because it demonstrates the IPAF's relevance across several interpersonal domains.

3. Working in the transference is essential *when the patient finds it difficult to report INs,* or is very isolated, and hence what transpires between the patient and therapist is effectively the most "live" material available to work with.

4. Taking up the transference can also be used to *reinforce the working alliance* when this is threatened by the activation in the patient's mind of negative feelings or unsettling fantasies about the therapist (e.g. if there seems to be a danger that the patient will drop out of therapy because the patient believes that the therapist wants to get rid of him). These may or may not be part of the chosen IPAF, but should be attended to nevertheless.

5. When the therapist considers that the INs reported by the patient are being used to create emotional distance from the IPAF (e.g. the pattern is something happening "out there"), a transference interpretation about what is going on in the here and now helps *to refocus the patient on his more immediate experience and the IPAF.*

Case example

Graham was in his mid-forties. He presented to his GP requesting help with his increasing unhappiness, his low self-esteem, and self-doubt. His personal and professional life was becoming difficult. He felt "old" and "fragile." The GP noted that he had experienced anxiety and depression for the last year, he was finding social situations difficult, and his libido had decreased.

On meeting Graham for the first time the therapist was struck by his physical appearance. He was very tall and seemed to tower over her in the waiting room. She had an immediate experience of feeling small. He was also thin and appeared awkward in his body, stooping in an attempt to reduce his height. He looked pale and slightly dishevelled and seemed young, dressed like a teenager. Also striking was his beaming smile. The smile conveyed hope and expectation. This smile became familiar to the therapist as Graham showed it at the beginning and end of every session.

In the first four sessions the therapist explored his relationships, past and present. Graham was the middle of three siblings. One sister was two years older than him, the other three years younger. His sisters did not feature much at all in his account of family life. His father was in banking, "not happy or successful."

Work-related stress permeated family life. Graham described his father as "objective" and as his harshest critic, displaying no physical affection or emotional support. He had felt like a constant disappointment to him. He reported that his father made attempts to hide his disappointment and displeasure by "objectivity," but Graham felt that he could easily "see through" this. His relationship with his mother, he said, was different. They were very close; there was nothing to hide. He felt he knew her so well he could anticipate her emotional state, especially when she was stressed and upset. Overall he felt that he had been experienced as a demanding and needy child. His grandfather had told him he would often make his mother cry because he was so demanding.

The therapist was interested to note that she did not experience Graham as demanding—quite the opposite. He was clearly anxious but did not challenge or question her. However, he did seem somewhat brittle and on his guard, which had an impact on the therapist; she felt anxious about intruding too much. She also felt that he was hiding the extent of his distress from her.

In this initial phase of the therapy Graham was very preoccupied with his body. Because of his height and thin physique he had always felt different from others and lacking in physical strength. He described this as feeling "wonky." He felt embarrassed by his body and mostly kept it covered up, even in hot weather. Sports activities as a child had been a cruel reminder of his "wonkiness" and he tried hard to avoid any kind of exercise as an adult. In his mind it became apparent that the trigger for his help seeking had been his perception of his failing body. The cracks were showing for all to see, he felt. He was experiencing aches and pains, which he saw as a confirmation of his ageing body. He said that he "hated feeling old."

Graham's interpersonal world was quite impoverished. He mentioned two or three important friends from the past, but no current ones. The most important relationship was with his partner. As Graham spoke about these relationships the therapist was able to see a clear pattern emerging: Graham was often left feeling very judged and criticized by the other person, just as he had felt by his father. This was beginning to emerge in the transference too. The therapist's countertransference was of note: she was beginning to feel that she needed to keep herself free of criticism from him, often feeling a pressure to "get things right." She monitored her use of words and her facial expression, as if alert to the possibility of criticizing him. She was able to explore this in the transference, illustrating to Graham how their relationship was suffused with his expectation that she would be crushing of him and that his very need for help was confirmation of his "wonkiness."

Through his narrative and her understanding of the evolving transference–countertransference, the therapist developed the following IPAF: Graham had a long-standing experience of a critical unaffectionate father who was unable to disguise his disappointment in him. He had grown up with the family "story" that his neediness made his mother cry. As a young child he began to anticipate his mother's moods. Importantly he began to develop a view of himself as demanding, inferior, and "wonky." His awkward body was a visual representation of his wonky self. He began to experience and expect others to be critical of this wonky self and to have no capacity for responding to his neediness, ultimately disappointing him. The IPAF that was agreed on focused on a "critical, judging" other representation and Graham's self-representation as "wonky and inferior," which triggered a feeling of depression and loneliness, as he then invariably withdrew from others.

Graham seemed to accept the IPAF. He responded to it by giving an example from his primary school days that helped the therapist to further fine tune the IPAF: he was trying to make a prop for the school play and was intent on making it the best in his class. He wasn't content with second best. His mother, seeing him struggle, offered to help. Graham said he had felt irritated and angry. He knew how he wanted it to be. It emerged that what had made him so angry was his belief that his mother would only succeed in making the prop the "same as everybody else's": ordinary. This was unbearable for two reasons. His need for help had been uncovered and there was an intention, so he felt, to reduce him to something ordinary and not special.

This story was explored in the transference. There was evidence that Graham had been anxious to know if he was the therapist's only patient, and she had increasingly experienced him as needing to be in a one-up position when he was beginning to feel vulnerable or criticized by her. She was reminded of her first meeting with him and her feeling of smallness. The therapist therefore took up in her eventual interpretation how Graham feared exposure of his need for her. Importantly the therapist began to understand that alongside Graham's view of himself as wonky and inferior, and hence his anticipation that the other might criticize him, there was another self-representation as someone special and superior.

Graham also described ways in which he avoided knowing about the ordinary aspects of his relationships and how he had a secret contempt for the prosaic. He often sabotaged experiences by reducing them to a cliché. As a teenager he had looked for something profound and special in his relationships. He also began to explore how his work as an academic had kept him in an elevated position. He had been in a special place as a student as he had been taken under the wing of a prominent professor. This had been an effective way of preserving his self-esteem until younger, more successful students came along to challenge his view of himself and left him feeling old.

The middle phase of therapy was spent looking at the loss and pain involved for Graham in facing his ordinariness, his neediness, the limitations of his aging, and the implications of this for his work. The elevated superior part of him needed help to accept that there may be things in life that he would never achieve and to free himself from the internal critical father figure that he had spent so much of his life relating to. The therapy also explored the consequences of keeping others at a distance. He was able to see that he was missing out on a lot of pleasure in his life. Graham was tempted to reduce the IPAF to a cliché—a "mid-life crisis," but he managed not to, and worked hard at challenging his familiar ways of being in relationships.

The therapist was able to anticipate that the ending would be difficult for Graham. It meant giving up on the idea of a "special" therapy, just for him. Exploring this in the transference was very important. It helped Graham to acknowledge his need for help, revealing more of his fragile and wonky self, which lay him open to feeling exposed.

The bridge to change

In longer-term psychotherapy the emphasis remains more firmly placed on work in the transference, and links to other current relationships are generally discouraged. In DIT, as we have been suggesting, the transference is actively used to help the patient to observe the manifestation of the IPAF in other current relationships so that it can be used as a "bridge" to supporting change. Whilst it would be clearly unhelpful to be prescriptive about the timing for this, in DIT there is a more explicit effort to help the patient to eventually extrapolate from the transference to his external world of relationships so as to support attempts at new ways of relating.

Case example

Sara—a young woman suffering from debilitating anxiety—struggled with therapy from the outset. This was largely on account of the fact that Sara felt she had to rely entirely on herself. This emerged as an expectation that had taken root early on in her life when she felt her parents to be emotionally unavailable to her. In her eighth session, Sara's anxiety scores revealed a further deterioration in her anxiety, which had in fact been worsening over several weeks.

The therapist invited Sara to tell her what she made of this. Sara discussed difficulties with her partner: she found it very hard to communicate to him what she needed from their relationship. She then talked generally about the bleakness of the future, how nothing could really change things, that her marriage was stuck, and that she was dreading raising with her husband the fact that she did not want to visit her in-laws over the forthcoming holidays. She wished she could just "magically disappear" so as to avoid this confrontation.

The therapist felt that Sara sounded distant and disconnected as she spoke. She experienced Sara as hopeless about the therapy, and thought to herself that the patient might not come back the following week—that she might "disappear" so as to avoid a more direct discussion about the therapy. The therapist eventually said:

> T: I think it would be helpful if we pause for a minute to look at what has just been happening here between us, because it seems to me that you are feeling rather despairing and hopeless about whether coming here can be of any

help to you, and your anxiety does seem to be getting worse, and yet you are not communicating this directly to me. Instead I feel you withdrawing. We know how difficult it is for you to be in the position of feeling that you are on your own with a problem and that the other person cannot help you with it. This often leaves you feeling angry, but instead of expressing what you feel you shut down communication. This is similar to what happens with your husband when you get into a conflict with him, just as you were describing to me earlier on in the session.

P: I know. I do that. I don't feel able to change this. I don't seem able to communicate normally with others. It must be frustrating for you . . .

T: What is difficult here is that you pull away instead of us being able to think together about how you are feeling worse and how you feel the therapy is not helping. The risk then is that you might just not come back, that you might disappear . . .

P: [Sounds taken aback] I have been thinking about whether it's worth continuing with this . . . I hadn't wanted to tell you though in case you thought I was being difficult.

T: So it's safer not to tell me, but this also then means that there is no possibility for us to work out a way forwards.

The therapist and patient were then able to unpack this impasse further, making it eventually also possible for the therapist to invite the patient to reflect on how she might approach the unspoken tension between her and her husband in relation to the dreaded stay with the in-laws. The therapist actively encouraged the patient to try to speak with her husband about it, just as she had managed to speak to her in the session.

If we unpack the therapist's first intervention, it reveals several components:

The *first step* is to "mark a moment" in the interpersonal exchange in the here and now and invite the patient to pause so as to reflect on it:

> I think it would be helpful if we pause for a minute to look at what has just been happening here between us . . .

The *second step* involves exploring the uncomfortable feelings that are not directly communicated:

> It seems to me that you are feeling rather despairing and hopeless about whether coming here can be of any help to you, and your anxiety does seem to be getting worse, and yet you are not communicating this directly to me.

The *third step* involves empathizing with and beginning to explore around the edges of the self–other representation that is being activated (i.e., the IPAF), which may reflect a particular defensive function:

> Instead I see you withdrawing and we know how difficult it is for you to be in the position of feeling that you are on your own with a problem and that the other person cannot help you with it. This often leaves you feeling angry but instead of expressing what you feel you shut down communication.

The *fourth step* involves linking the transference pattern to other current interpersonal contexts that are being focused on in the therapy:

> This is so similar to what happens with your husband when you get into a conflict with him, just as you were describing to me earlier on in the session . . .

This *final step* marks the invitation to work on a current interpersonal issue as the therapist and patient indeed went on to do in this case.

Chapter 9

When Things Go Wrong

Managing difficulties in the therapeutic relationship

No matter how well trained or how much personal therapy we have undertaken, some of the time, we all get it wrong. This "getting it wrong" may have different sources and meanings. It may indicate a momentary lapse in attentiveness, for example, which says more about our state of mind than being the result of the patient's projections. There are also those occasions when things go "wrong" because we are drawn into an enactment, responding to unconscious pressure from the patient to behave in particular ways that resonate with the IPAF.

Some patients need to "test" the relationship with the therapist in the transference. For example, we may need to stand the test of the patient's hostility or of their mistrust. Sometimes, we will find ourselves behaving towards the patient just as he anticipated. Such experiences, however difficult for us, require careful processing, rather than being "batted back" through a premature interpretation, which might leave the patient feeling that we cannot tolerate his feelings towards us.

A classical analytic position presumes the analyst's capacity for objectivity, and so neutrality, thus bestowing upon the therapist a privileged status about knowing or discovering a hidden "truth" about the patient. The therapist is seen to be an objective presence interpreting to a subjectively distorting, unrealistic, self-deceiving patient. Increasingly, however, therapists from diverse schools of psychoanalysis recognize that, for the most part, unconscious processes govern the patient–therapist interaction. Notions of neutrality then become problematic and, along with abstinence and anonymity—the classical triad emblematic of the analytic stance—they appear antithetical to the unavoidable mutual interaction at work in the patient–therapist dyad.

Notwithstanding significant theoretical and technical differences on this point, there is nevertheless a fair degree of consensus that enactments by the therapist are an unavoidable reality as the therapist is a participant in the analytic process (see for example Steiner, 2000). Recognizing their inevitability (by the patient, therapist, or both) is a basic starting point for any therapist.

Reflective practice: monitoring the countertransference

At their best the patient and therapist strive together to be observers of the states of mind that emerge during the course of a therapy so that these can be reflected upon, but since we are frequently pulled away from an analytic stance by factors in both the patient and in ourselves, the work of therapy relies on our capacity to reestablish this reflective stance.

Working in the transference involves recognizing our countertransference and making use of it to add to the formulation, moment by moment, of the transference. We attend to the specific quality of the feelings, thoughts, flow of associations, and fantasies that are evoked in us during the exchanges with the patient so as to hypothesize about what the patient may be expressing indirectly. We underline, once again, that it is a *hypothesis*, not necessarily a fact, because it is easy to equate one's own emotional conviction (e.g. "I felt so angry as I listened to the patient and I think this is what she cannot bear to know in herself") with the reality of the patient's state of mind. The countertransference is an important source of information, as rich in the insights it can facilitate as it is in the possibilities it also offers us for misattributing states of mind to the patient that, in fact, belong to us. This is because the countertransference is a complex phenomenon and consequently it can be misused: in this sense the countertransference is the best of servants, but the worst of masters (Segal, 1993).

As we define it here the countertransference consists of three dimensions: the therapist's ordinary emotional response to the patient's predicament, the therapist's own transference to the patient, and the patient's projections into the therapist, which give rise to emotional responses in the therapist. All three dimensions need to be borne in mind when trying to understand the therapist's feelings or fantasies so that it becomes part of routine practice to critically consider the meaning of the therapist's emotional reactions to the patient. This way we can minimize the risk of unsubstantiated speculation or of misattributing to the patient feelings that belong to us.

In order to make use of our responsiveness to the patient as the basis for interpretation, we have to reflect on our involvement in the therapeutic process in the context of the rapid shifts that can occur in the patient's states of mind (and that sometimes recruit us into taking up highly specified roles in relation to the patient). The therapeutic process relies on our ability to be open to experiencing transitory identifications with the patient's projections through allowing the patient to view us in a manner incongruent with our own self-perception, so as to understand the meaning of this for the patient (i.e., not interpreting this prematurely).

Maintaining an "observing distance" from the part of us that is involved in the process is best facilitated through regular discussion of cases with peers or supervisors. This is especially important when learning a new way of doing things: the anxiety normally associated with demonstrating competence in the new model not uncommonly results in clinicians so preoccupied with "doing it right" that in the process they neglect basic therapeutic skills they are familiar with and experienced in. In other words, under these circumstances, the potential for enactments is enhanced.

Enactments, as we have been suggesting, are not only inevitable, but also potentially helpful as long as we can process their meaning and use the understanding gleaned to further the therapy. Being drawn into an enactment gives us first-hand experience of what happens in the patient's relationships. But some enactments may lead to the violation of boundaries that damage the work and the patient, and hence we need to be vigilant and monitor ourselves. We can never justify an enactment that breaches ethical boundaries even if on account of the interactional pressures placed on the therapist by the patient. Patients may well want to transform us into all kinds of different objects, but we always remain, in reality, a therapist who must practice within professional boundaries.

Therapeutic stance when managing misunderstandings and misattunements in the therapist–patient relationship

Like any relationship, the therapeutic relationship can suffer the strains of misunderstandings and misattunements. When they do occur, we approach this with an "open to correction" stance that signals to the patient that we are prepared to examine what may have gone wrong in a nondefensive manner. The critical part of the process is to slow the discourse down so that the misapprehension can be explored fully and carefully. Approaching these difficulties with interest in the patient's experience of the therapist, committed to identifying and taking responsibility for the respective roles of patient and therapist in contributing to the problem that has arisen, implicitly models a mentalizing stance. Where appropriate, we recognize and acknowledge our contribution to the patient's response. For example, a therapist yawned and the patient reacted with anger. In exploring this, the therapist acknowledged that she had yawned and that this had been felt to be provocative by the patient, inviting him then to think about what the yawn signaled to him.

If we have somehow contributed to the patient's experience through an enactment this needs exploration too. This is important because a major aspect of working in the transference is to model a capacity for reflecting on what happens in relationships, which involves acknowledging mistakes or misunderstandings. Acknowledging our "mistake" does not require, however, explaining why we made the mistake: this is the patient's therapy, not ours. But it *is* important to acknowledge that we did something that ideally we should not have done, that this had an impact on the patient, and that we are keen to understand this.

The patient's conscious and unconscious fantasies, for example, about the cause of a therapist's temporary lapse in attentiveness would then become the focus of joint exploration of the patient's conviction that this was due to how boring he is. It is important for the therapist to be open about the way her own mind works. This engenders curiosity as well as creating motivation for adopting alternative perspectives. This stance is important for several reasons. The acknowledgement of an error models honesty and courage. In taking responsibility for the "error" or a behavior felt to be provocative in some way by the patient, this also tends to lower the patient's arousal. Finally it also offers an opportunity to revisit how such scenarios arise out of mistaken assumptions about opaque mental states and how misunderstanding can lead to aversive experiences.

The therapeutic relationship is strengthened by the experience of difficulties that can be openly discussed and resolved. Misunderstandings and ruptures in the therapeutic relationship allow the therapist to model how to manage interpersonal conflict, and how to disentangle the intentions and attitudes of those involved.

Case example

Ms A., a rather brittle young woman, had always felt herself to be in the shadow of her older and seemingly more successful sister. She had comforted herself with being the "good daughter" who had stayed close to her parents and taken care of them in their old age.

The IPAF that was agreed on centered on her recurring experience of feeling herself to be "undesirable" relating to an object that was felt to be "preoccupied and unavailable" to her. This invariably gave rise to depressed affect that paralysed her. Her recent depression had followed the sudden death of her mother and she had then struggled to manage taking care of her father whose grief and pining for his wife left Ms A. feeling that her care and attention were "insufficient." She spoke about her mother as a very engaging, funny woman whom the father loved and admired. It felt to the therapist that Ms A. had hoped that she could somehow replace her mother in her father's affections, and that she could finally be the one who was desired. The father's seemingly entrenched grief, however, was interpreted by Ms A. as the painful, if all too familiar, confirmation that she was simply not desirable enough. The object, as far as she was concerned, always had a more desirable "other" in mind.

In session seven the therapist and patient agreed to change the time of the next session at the therapist's behest. The following week the patient turned up at the correct "new" time, but the therapist was not there—she had, in fact, got confused and was expecting the patient the following day. When she later realized her mistake, the therapist had then written to the patient to apologize for the confusion.

When they finally met again, Ms A. was late and the therapist felt her to be hostile. Even before the therapist could say anything about the previous week's events, the patient began to speak in a very pressured manner. The therapist thought that Ms A. was desperately suppressing her rage. The patient spoke about her disappointment with the therapy and with the therapist:

> P: It's not as though I had high expectations . . . that would have been unreasonable, and no-one knows how this verbal therapy works . . . perhaps medication is better, I read that somewhere . . . I don't know . . . I wish I had not

embarked on this . . . you said it was important to attend all sessions . . . the importance of not losing momentum . . . at the very least I had expected I would be treated with respect, not treated like a "second-class" citizen who can't even rely on being seen at the right time . . . It was so embarrassing being in reception in front of other patients and being told your therapist is not there . . . they were all looking at me . . . glaring as if there was something odd about me.

T: It was entirely my confusion that led to you being left stranded without a session last week, and exposed to the harsh glare of the other patients, and as I said in my letter, I am sorry about this. It is understandable that you should feel upset about it and unsettled by this especially since I have been so emphatic about the importance of attending sessions.

The patient visibly calmed down at this point. The therapist then went on, trying to link the "event" in the therapy to the IPAF:

T: I think that it would nevertheless be helpful to think together about what has made my mistake feel so upsetting in this very particular kind of way because what strikes me about your experience in the reception area is how you felt harshly scrutinized by the other patients. It wasn't only that I was not there, but that you then felt my absence exposed something unappealing about you.
P: [The patient nodded] It felt just awful . . .
T: Awful . . .
P: I mean, ashamed, like I wanted to dig a hole and disappear and then also angry, furious, like I was about to explode . . . incensed . . . that's what I felt—I could both believe that this was happening to me—because these things *always* happen to me—and at the same time I felt incensed.
T: I think that your connection with the feelings of shame followed by outrage is important. My not being here for you last week cast you right back in that painful familiar role of being the undesirable, insufficient one who is not kept in mind—instead someone else gets the attention you so desperately feel you need and is due to you—and I think this is what you imagined the other patients could see. And you sway from feeling ashamed and then feeling outraged, that it's unfair . . .
P: When I was told by the receptionist that you were not there I felt at first that I was to blame—I always feel that even though I knew I had the right time in my diary. Still I thought the receptionist must have got it wrong . . .
T: So at that moment you were still holding on to some hope that this could not be happening, that you had got it right and that I would also get it right and appear, as I should have done.
P: Yes, exactly, but as time passed and you did not pitch up I started to feel really angry towards you. It was like a wave of rage, which I felt still as I got here today . . .
T: Rage towards me for not being there . . . where did you think I was?

P: I was convinced that another patient had called in, someone with more important, interesting issues than the crap I repeat every week, and that you just offered to see them instead of me.

T: So the rage you felt then and are still feeling today has something to do with me becoming in your experience someone who actively neglects you because you are not as interesting as the patient you think I chose to see instead of you . . .

The patient's elaboration of her fantasy about the reason for the therapist's forgetting provided an immediate opportunity to help the patient observe the activation of the IPAF in the transference.

Irrespective of what motivated the therapist's confusion in the first place, this incident became an important landmark in the work, which gave Ms A. greater confidence in her therapist's ability to tolerate her rage and reinforced the relevance of the IPAF. The therapist's ordinary openness about her error was an important precondition for this development because it modeled a way of taking responsibility for something that had gone wrong and for how conflict can be resolved.

It is easier for patients to give voice to negative feelings if they trust that the therapist can tolerate their expression without retaliating or trying to minimize their significance. As was the case with Ms A., responding to such feelings requires that the therapist is able to critically scrutinize her own contribution to any difficulties or impasses in the relationship.

Forms of resistance

In the therapeutic situation defenses manifest themselves as resistances, which undermine the conscious contract the therapist and patient have signed up to. The term resistance means essentially opposition. Resistance can take many forms. It refers to any defensive maneuver, as deployed in the therapeutic situation, which impedes the therapeutic work. It signals an avoidance of unsettling feelings or thoughts by the patient that is subjectively experienced by the therapist as being somehow drawn away from the agreed focus. Resistances can be "obvious," for example, when the patient arrives late, or they can be "unobtrusive" (Glover, 1955), as when the patient appears compliant but the compliance masks hostility to the process.

Because resistance occurs in the context of the therapeutic relationship it is incumbent on us to acknowledge the "external" triggers that may compound a resistance, for example, cancellations by the therapist.

It is also very important to differentiate resistances from the patient's disagreement with us: the patient's "No" sometimes does mean just that.

Starting therapy always represents a threat to the patient's emotional status quo. The early stages of DIT are thus ripe for resistances of various sorts because the patient's anxiety about beginning therapy will be very active and has not yet been sufficiently reflected upon with the therapist for that process to provide sufficient containment.

To understand resistance we need to think about the different, and all too often conflicting, motivations that lie beneath the patient's resolve to seek help. In other words, we need to consider the patient's relationship to help and its internal meaning. Suffering often acts as a spur to seeking help, but not invariably. For every wish to be helped we often find the converse wish, within the same patient, to maintain the status quo due, for example, to the threat of the therapy to the patient's self-esteem or the patient's need to keep the pain alive (i.e., secondary gain). Often the patient wants to both get better *and* stay the same. Some patients are more fundamentally "against understanding" (Joseph, 1983: 139) and these patients are highly unlikely to benefit from DIT.

The patient's relationship to help is organized around procedures for being helped that have most probably been set in early childhood. Such procedures will be activated when beginning therapy and will become known to us in the transference (and this is what we often aim to capture when we listen to "cautionary tales"—see Chapter 4). Enquiring at the assessment stage into the patient's previous experiences of therapy or relationships with other healthcare professionals, friends, and family will enrich our formulation and help us to anticipate particular difficulties in engaging with the therapeutic process.

It is beyond the scope of this book to cover all possible forms of resistance exhaustively. This section is therefore restricted to describing those common scenarios encountered especially, but not exclusively, in the initial stages of DIT, and which may act as a form of resistance.

Requests for information about DIT

It is important for the patient to have information about DIT in order to meaningfully consent to it. Answering some of his questions about it is therefore part of good clinical practice. For some patients, however, these questions are pregnant with meaning that goes well beyond the need to have some idea of what the patient is agreeing to. In such a scenario the therapist might say:

> Beginning psychotherapy can make people feel anxious because it is frightening and painful to confront certain aspects of oneself. I'm wondering if asking me a lot of practical questions is perhaps your way of letting me know that you are worried about what you are letting yourself in for?

In the vast majority of cases taking up the anxiety behind the question is enough to ease the patient into therapy.

Personal questions about the therapist

Many therapists struggle with how to manage requests by the patient for information about themselves (e.g. about the therapist's age, culture, or family circumstances). On the face of it some of these questions may seem reasonable, and the therapist may fear that by choosing not to answer the question this will create awkwardness in the interaction.

There is, of course, natural curiosity about the kind of person the therapist is, but this apparent curiosity is often multilayered and may serve a range of defensive functions that require understanding. For this reason self-disclosure of personal information about the therapist is discouraged in DIT. Instead, it is more productive to approach such requests by acknowledging the importance of the question to the patient and then inviting him to be curious about "what else" he may trying to communicate/ask for.

Having said this, when these questions arise in the first sessions we need to balance exploration with engaging the patient in the therapy. For those patients not acculturated to a psychodynamic mode of working, not answering such questions may seem odd. We need to ensure that in remaining true to our "model" we don't shame or alienate the patient. In a response to a question, for example, about whether the therapist has children, the therapist might preface the invitation to explore what may lie behind the question by saying something like:

> I appreciate that this is an important question for you and that my not answering it may seem odd to you, but I am interested to understand in what way might it make a difference to you if you knew whether I have children or not?

Now, if this question about children was posed by a patient who had been unable to conceive children, the question, we might hypothesize, is emotionally loaded given such a history and would have a particular poignancy. The therapist might then say:

> I can imagine that this is a really important question for you given what you have been struggling with in your own life. You may well be wondering how I could understand your loss if I have children ...

Requests for direction/advice

Generally speaking, direct advice is proscribed in DIT (except, for example, if the patient is suicidal and action needs to be taken to ensure safety, or if the patient may require a referral on to another professional). Requests for advice are not uncommon, however, in the early stages of DIT, especially from patients who know little about how psychotherapy works and who consequently base their expectations of it on the model they are most familiar with, namely the medical model where advice is given liberally. The patient's cultural background may also be relevant in this respect: in cultures where psychotherapy is not common and where the expectation is that the "doctor" gives pills or advice, requests for advice are best addressed first by explaining the nature of psychotherapy and then dealing with how the patient feels about this. For example the therapist might say:

> I can see that in coming here you expected me to give you advice and practical suggestions to help you with your difficulties. I wonder what it feels like to discover that I am a different kind of therapist to the one you had expected.

In some cases the request for advice may betray the patient's wish for an idealized therapist who is omnipotent and will cure them of his ills, or it may reveal the patient's characteristic passive stance in relation to his problems. Here it will therefore be important to take this up with the patient and to articulate the possible meaning.

Challenging the boundaries of the therapeutic relationship

Patients can use the therapeutic frame as the focus of their resistance, for example, by coming late or trying to extend sessions. Requests for contact in between sessions may represent yet another means of challenging the boundaries of the therapeutic frame. It would be meaningless to try to anticipate the meanings such behavior may have since it will be specific to the individual patient, but often such challenges to the therapeutic frame are a call to the therapist to take these up in the transference.

The IPAF as an intellectual defense against feeling

Patients come into therapy in search of answers. Some patients, however, convey an urgent need to be relieved of their symptoms and the uncertainty that "not knowing" can give rise to. This anxiety may be managed by a retreat into a search for certainty. For such a patient the IPAF may provide the kind of certainty they are seeking and the formulation is therefore enthusiastically welcomed, but soon the therapist is left feeling that no real contact can be made with the patient, that the links to the IPAF are superficial and nothing changes. Here the use made of the IPAF becomes the focus of exploration.

The compliant patient

It is not uncommon for patients to project their own critical superegos into us so that we are then experienced as judgmental or punitive. When this occurs the patient may retreat into compliance and will try to say or do the right thing so as to please us and avoid our disapproval. He may agree with the IPAF, dutifully bring examples each week that confirm it, and the therapist may be pleased with the progress. And yet there is a little change in the patient's life. In so doing the patient is resisting the process since he is not able to examine this dynamic, something that might, in turn, expose him to his own more critical, hostile feelings towards the therapist. The problem for the therapist in these cases is that it is all too easy to fall into the comfortable trap of being in therapy with the patient who is always nice, appreciative, and interested but who simply does not change because we collude with his defense.

Difficulty in being the patient

One way of avoiding exploring oneself and of denying feelings of vulnerability or dependency is to defend against being a patient. Rationalizing, intellectualizing, or acting seductively may all be deployed as a means of avoiding vulnerability. Such patients may be very adept at drawing us into intellectual—and often very stimulating—discussions, which nevertheless serve the function of abolishing any differences between the therapist and the patient so that his vulnerability is avoided.

Idealizing the therapist

The DIT therapist makes the most of the positive transference, when it is accessible, in order to engage the patient and drive the therapy forwards. She does so mindful that this will likely give way to the negative transference, some of the time. A positive transference is, however, quite different to an idealized one and reliably gives way to denigration.

Given our own narcissistic needs it may be difficult to resist the pull of the patient who thinks we are wonderful (though it helps if we remind ourselves that idealization is invariably followed by denigration). The patient may need to think we are wonderful because any other thoughts and feelings might be too threatening. If we become too identified with being a "wonderful" therapist, we will not be able to stand back and help the patient think about what idealization defends against.

Sexualized behavior

Sexualization of the therapeutic relationship is often used as a means of resisting feelings of vulnerability or powerlessness. Seduction can be quite explicitly erotized or it may be more subtle and therefore even more difficult to grasp. A subtle form of seduction, for example, can be observed in the way some patients disclose information: some patients tell their story enigmatically or very colorfully and we find ourselves gripped by the story, wanting to hear more. Often this reflects the patient's attempt to draw us out of our interpretative function through seducing us. Again, this is a call for the therapist's self-reflection.

The therapist's resistance to time-limited work

It is not just the patient who may engage half-heartedly in the therapy. The therapist, too, can bring into play her own resistances. We have in mind here, more specifically, the resistance to time-limited work.

In order to work in any therapeutic modality the therapist needs to feel that she is delivering a therapy that has integrity and that is felt to be potentially beneficial to the patient. DIT is no exception, but its delivery may pose particular problems to practitioners who are very committed to long-term, open-ended therapy and who may consequently feel they are somehow short-changing the patient if they offer sixteen sessions.

In our experience it is not uncommon for the therapist to present what she is offering the patient in exactly these terms: "We will meet for *only* sixteen sessions." Our prejudices about brief therapy may well leak through and convey to the patient that what he is being offered falls short of what he needs. Of course, with some patients, this will indeed be the case, and it will be important to help the patient to express his own experience of disappointment as well as the therapist's.

However, when trained in long-term therapy, it may also be difficult to imagine that sixteen sessions could be enough time to help a patient to make some important changes, or that for some patients this may be all that they can manage at a given point in time. It is therefore incumbent on all of us to examine our own belief systems in this respect so as to be freed of unhelpful assumptions that may set up the therapeutic encounter to fail.

Working with resistance

The first stage of working with resistance requires a formulation of the patient's relationship to help: that is, we strive to make sense of what internal object relationship is activated when the patient experiences himself as needy and vulnerable in relation to us as the helper. This may or may not be relevant to the IPAF, but if the patient is resistant to being helped, then this becomes the therapeutic priority.

Many resistances, as we mentioned earlier, emerge specifically in relation to the anticipation of receiving help. For example, a patient whose experience of being vulnerable had become equated early on with being humiliated found it intolerable to take in anything the therapist offered him because he experienced his "not-knowing" (which he equated with being the patient) as deeply humiliating. He therefore met all interpretations with contempt, making the therapist feel like the "stupid" one who always got it wrong. This internalized object relationship got in the way of him being able to derive help from the therapy and hence had to be addressed.

Once we have grasped the quality of the patient's relationship to help we can begin to reflect on whether the patient "won't" accept help or "can't" accept help. This distinction relates to the important consideration of whether the resistance results from an internal conflict or from a deficit. The greater the degree of personality integration typically associated with a neurotic personality structure, the more likely it will be that the resistance arises from a conflict between a part of the patient that wants help and another that finds some substitute satisfaction in maintaining the symptoms.

The less integrated patient may, on the contrary, be resisting help because to allow another person into his world is simply experienced as too dangerous. This is the kind of patient who feels that he cannot afford to take the risk to allow the therapist into his world. In his history we often encounter developmental deficits. Our task here is to find ways of communicating that we understand what the experience of being in therapy might feel like for the patient. This patient, for instance, may have a template for being helped that involves an abusive other masquerading as a helper. In such an instance, the therapist strives to convey respect for the defensive structure that has protected the patient and names the feared risks of letting the therapist into his world.

Working with resistance is approached in the same way as we suggest approaching defenses (see Chapter 6), that is gradually and through building up to an interpretation once the patient has first been helped to acknowledge that he is not allowing himself to be helped (Greenson, 1967) (see Figure 9.1). For example, say the patient has been arriving late for a few sessions and that this is occurring in the latter part of the middle phase, that is, as the therapy is inching closer to the endings. The therapist would go through the following steps before making an interpretation:

- The therapist begins by pointing out to the patient that he is resisting using unambiguous examples of why she thinks this: "It's the third time you arrived late this month and I think this is perhaps not just accidental."

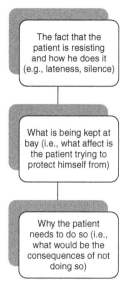

Figure 9.1 Steps for interpreting resistance in the therapeutic relationship.

- The therapist then invites the patient to be curious about the meaning of his behavior before making an interpretation: "Do you have any thoughts about this?"

- The patient may or may not provide any response to this. Either way the therapist tries to develop her understanding through both what the patient says and/or what he unconsciously conveys. In particular she formulates the affects the patient needs to protect himself from before interpreting the content of the resistance: "You seem to feel quite anxious in the sessions of late. I wonder if when you arrive so late, at least you feel in control of what happens here between us?"

- The final step is to make a fuller interpretation that takes into account the unconscious meaning of the resistance and links it to the IPAF where relevant: "It seems as though, since I brought up the ending a few weeks ago, you have found it very hard to arrive on time. I am wondering if my reminder felt like me pushing you away. We know from the work we have been doing that when you feel this way in your relationships you withdraw and can actually start to do the rejecting—I think this may be what has been happening here: you come late and I am the one waiting here, the one who is left out, not knowing whether I have a patient or not."

In this chapter, we have reviewed the different kinds of therapeutic challenges that may arise in the course of the therapeutic encounter. We hope that we have conveyed that exploring what happens in the transference is very important when there is a need to explore difficulties in the therapy, but as we saw in Chapter 8, its use is more circumscribed than is the case in other psychodynamic models, as it is informed by whether it supports the two central strategies in DIT: exploring the IPAF and helping the patient to better understand his mental states.

Chapter 10

The Ending Phase

The focus on the importance of attachments means that in DIT the separation from the therapist is regarded as an important event. The last four sessions are therefore devoted to an exploration of the conscious and unconscious meaning for the patient of ending the therapy and to reflecting on the work that has been achieved. In this chapter we will review the aims and strategies of the *ending phase*.

The patient's response to endings

At the core of psychodynamic accounts about the significance of ending therapy lies the assumption that endings restimulate other salient experiences of separation such as bereavements, transitions (e.g. leaving home), or the ending of other significant relationships.

Each patient reacts differently but, generally speaking, ending therapy elicits feelings of loss as well as mobilizing anxiety about separation. These feelings are not always expressed directly. One of our tasks in the ending phase is to help the patient to articulate his feelings about ending. This requires us to closely monitor and respond to his experience in order to minimize the likelihood of premature endings or other enactments during this phase, which are typically associated with a difficulty in processing the experience of ending.

For many patients, endings force upon them the reality of separateness—an awareness that may be especially challenging for some. In one sense the end of every session is a separation, which is why the end of sessions often provides opportunities for acting out (e.g. the patient who seemingly ignores that the therapist has called time). The end of each session can feel like an unwelcome reminder that therapist and patient are two separate beings. As the therapist calls time the patient, depending on his own experiences, hears and feels different things: he may feel rejected or abandoned or humiliated. For those patients who experience separation in this manner, the final ending of therapy only serves to accentuate further these feelings and the associated fantasies.

For some patients the briefness of DIT may "dull" some of the feelings that longer-term and more intensive therapy typically accentuates because the person of the therapist becomes a very central attachment figure over a long period of time. Yet clinical experience typically illustrates that even over a period of sixteen sessions, many patients develop intense feelings towards the therapist. For example, for some patients, the very briefness of the encounter may mobilize an intense transference in which the therapist is experienced as tantalizingly seductive and cruel, inviting then into an intimacy only to then leave them. Moreover, precisely *because* of the brevity of the therapy, such feelings can emerge in a more intense manner because the patient cannot "push to one side" in his own mind the experience of separation as it is clearly present from the outset.

How the patient is able to end the therapy encapsulates his level of psychological functioning at the time and, in many cases, is a good indicator of how the patient has progressed in therapy. This is because ending "well" (that is, in a way that allows for the expression of disappointment, loss, and gratitude) involves a number of related processes:

◆ *Ending entails mourning.* The work of mourning requires of the patient that he can relate to the therapist as a whole object with imperfections without this overshadowing the strengths or qualities that will also be missed. Ending requires accepting the separateness of the therapist and the pain that this can give rise to. Working through this loss promotes internalization of the therapeutic relationship. This then allows the patient to establish the therapeutic process as a structure within his mind: that is, the patient becomes self-reflective. This internalization can only occur once the patient has accepted the therapist's separateness and mourned the loss.

◆ *Ending involves re-owning projections.* Over the course of therapy the therapist often becomes the container of the patient's projections—a repository for the split-off aspects of the self. Ending involves relinquishing this container as the patient has to re-own what belongs to him and learn to bear it within himself.

- *Ending requires relinquishing sole possession of the therapist.* It involves coming to terms with being replaced by the next patient. This requires that the patient manages the feelings of envy and rivalry this may arouse without recourse to destructive attacks that devalue the therapeutic experience in the patient's mind, thereby allowing him to defensively come to terms with its loss.

Preparing for ending

As with any brief therapy, in practice, endings are not a discrete phase even if for the sake of clarity here we set it out as such. Rather, they are worked on from the start as the patient is reminded regularly of the brevity of the treatment. The therapist will be attuned, from the outset, to direct and indirect references to termination/separations. Throughout she will keep in mind, and help the patient to reflect on, the meaning of the time frame of therapy. This will be more or less relevant depending on the patient. In other words, the patient's history of loss and separation, which will invariably emerge as we sketch out the interpersonal map, will alert us to whether ending is likely to be challenging and in what way. It isn't so for all patients, however. We also need to recognize that, for those patients for whom separation is not a major psychological challenge, we don't need a sledgehammer to crack a nut: that is, we may not need to do the same kind of work around endings with all patients.

There are two core strategies for preparing the patient for ending and these are actively used from the start (Box 10.1). From a purely practical point of view, as we saw in Chapter 4, we contract with the patient a set number of sessions at the start, and we frequently make reference to the number of sessions left. This need not be every week necessarily, but once the middle phase work is underway, every few weeks it is helpful to refer to the number of sessions left. We also prepare the patient through drawing his attention to his subjective experience of separations as they occur in the context of the therapy, and in his life.

For those patients for whom endings are difficult, we may be put under pressure to extend the therapy (and hence avoid facing the ending). Here the therapist needs to maintain the boundary created by the time-limited nature of the therapy and help the patient to explore

Box 10.1 Ending phase strategies

- Encourage the patient to express affect related to ending
- Normalize the experience of anger, sadness, and loss if the patient is struggling to express his feelings
- Interpret the defensive aspects of denigrating or idealizing the therapy and you as the ending nears
- Systematically draw attention to, and address, the patient's feelings, fantasies, and anxieties about the ending of therapy
- Respond to the indications of regression near the end of treatment (e.g. a symptomatic deterioration) by linking this with the feelings and fantasies associated with endings
- Help the patient review the therapy as a whole (e.g. whether he has achieved his aims, whether the attachment style descriptions that the patient had selected have changed)
- Offer a "goodbye" letter which reviews the original agreed formulation and what progress has been made in working on the issues identified at the outset
- Help the patient express gratitude and/or disappointment, as appropriate

what the ending means to him. Such exploration may well start before session thirteen if we consider that the patient will find the ending especially challenging. As always we are guided by what the patient as an individual brings, rather than following the manual to the letter.

Although the ending will therefore always be in our mind, it is only in the last four sessions that there is an increasing, specific focus on the experience of ending. We will be especially alert to the opportunity during the ending phase of treatment to revisit the IPAF that has been worked on in the therapy. Not infrequently it sheds helpful light on why the patient may find the ending difficult.

Interpreting the unconscious meaning of endings

The particular emotional coloring that the ending assumes will vary considerably between patients depending on their unique developmental histories. The fact that the patient knows about the ending from the out-set does little to avert the fantasies that are often activated as the ending approaches. No matter how amenable or even positive the patient's con-scious response to the ending, it is best not to be seduced by it. It will always be closer to the truth to anticipate a mixed response, even when the work has gone well and the patient has made gains.

Some patients become very preoccupied in their own minds with the end. In these cases an important strategy in the ending phase is therefore to identify the unconscious fantasy that the patient has about why the therapy is coming to an end (Box 10.2). These fantasies mostly concern the patient's view of the therapist's mind and her perceived intentions in relation to him. In other words, they reflect the patient's experience of himself in relation to his object. Broadly speaking the fantasies are of two kinds, each respectively linked to more or less borderline/psychotic or neurotic levels of personality organization (this list should not be considered as exhaustive):

Paranoid and manic fantasies

♦ *Paranoid fantasies* reveal how the therapist is experienced as malevolently or ruthlessly leaving the patient behind because she no longer wants to see him. In these cases the patient's own hostility about ending is projected into the therapist who is then experienced as the one who is harming him by leaving. (This goes beyond what may be a reality, that the therapist has imposed the

Box 10.2 Preparing for ending

♦ Make contracts clear and specific at the outset
♦ Work with the ending from the start—keep referring to it in each session, if necessary, as a reminder from the middle phase onwards and explore the patient's reactions to this systematically
♦ Think about whether there are particular features of the patient's background and experiences that might make him especially sensitive to endings

time limit and the patient would like/benefit from more.
The feeling is one of being treated cruelly or hatefully.)

♦ *Manic fantasies* reflect the operation of primitive defensive
maneuvers to manage the ending (a) by attributing to the
therapist a sense of failure and incompetence (e.g. the patient
who views the ending as proof of the therapist's inability to
manage him), (b) by retreating into an omnipotent denial of her
significance in his life (e.g. the patient who denies any feelings of
loss and diminishes or by devaluing her helpfulness in his own
mind), or (c) by manically praising the therapist (gratitude that
has a false, controlling quality) creating the fantasy that the
therapist is one's own creation.

Neurotic fantasies

Neurotic fantasies are of two kinds:

♦ *Depressed fantasies* reveal the patient's preoccupation about his
impact on the therapist, for example, a fantasy that she is ending
the work—or at the very least not discouraging him from
ending—because she finds the patient boring or too demanding.

♦ *Oedipal fantasies* reveal the patient's preoccupation with "who
else" occupies the therapist's mind and who else is experienced as
more loveable, interesting, or exciting than he is. Two
qualitatively different fantasies have an oedipal flavor. In one
version the therapist is thought to be ending the therapy because
she has a more special patient in mind. In the second version she
is ending because there is another patient who needs her more
(e.g. "I understand we have to stop. There are more needy people
than me"). The latter reflects a defensive approach to the
existence of the rival—it is a defensive "giving up" of one's space
to an "other," which usually masks resentment.

Premature and prolonged endings

We offer sixteen sessions, but the patient may well decide to have fewer
sessions. Such decisions always deserve exploration in order to identify the conscious and unconscious factors that may be influencing
such a decision. Although a premature ending may well reflect the
patient's way of managing the anticipated ending, or it represents an

enactment of the IPAF, or it simply expresses the patient's difficulty in staying with the IPAF, we cannot assume that this is always the case. It is also important to explore nondefensively the possibility that DIT and/or the therapist's style are not felt to be helpful. Equally some patients may not require sixteen sessions and we need to be open to this possibility too.

At the other end of the spectrum we will encounter the patient who struggles to end and tries to prolong the therapy, for example, through repeated cancellations. This is one reason why we advise therapists to make it clear at the outset that the therapy is sixteen sessions long, to offer a clear outline of the schedule of sessions with planned breaks, and to explain that sessions are not automatically replaced. These are only guidelines and each therapist, partly depending on the service context and the protocols in place for missed sessions, may need to modify these guidelines. The main point is to ensure that there are some structures in place that help the therapist to stick to offering DIT over sixteen weekly sessions, in close succession rather than over a protracted period of time. This is important because when working briefly the momentum of the work is maintained partly through the continuity of sessions. The focus on change can easily be diluted by irregular sessions.

Ending: the therapist's perspective

Endings pose a challenge not only to the patient but also to the therapist. Just as our patients make an investment in us, and develop an attachment to us, so do we have an emotional investment in the therapeutic process and in the patient's life.

Endings are a time when not only the patient reviews his progress but also we assess our helpfulness or otherwise. If the patient has improved we vicariously partake in his achievement and we experience satisfaction in our work. Some patients will leave us feeling we have done a good job, while others leave us feeling we have failed and should start looking for an alternative career. Sometimes the sense of failure we experience can be understood as an attack by the patient, that is, his defense against loss: we become in the patient's mind a failed, useless object whose loss becomes trivial, thus easing the pain of separation.

In some cases we have to recognize that, unfortunately, we do fail our patients. This can be painful to bear. Some so-called failures are avoidable, but we have in mind here too the more ordinary failures that are unavoidable because no matter how good we are as a therapist, we can never be more than "good enough." Moreover, therapy can never hope to "correct" the deprivations some of our patients have suffered. It can offer understanding of the past, but it can never undo it. What we recognize rationally to be the limits of therapy can nevertheless be experienced by some patients as our personal failure towards them.

Because endings are infused with ambivalence, at the risk of sounding ungrateful, it is important to approach the patient's gratitude at the end of a therapy with curiosity to begin with rather than take it at face value. Hopefully, most of our patients are genuinely grateful to us for the help they have received. Gratitude is rooted in a realistic appraisal that therapy has not been a magic cure and that we are not all-wonderful but the patient still feels that we have offered something helpful. With some patients, however, the conscious expression of gratitude is excessive: we are talked about as "saviors" or as the parent they never had. As we approach endings we need to beware the seduction of idealization as much as the danger of denigration. Neither position will help our patients to deal with the infinitely more difficult psychic task of saying goodbye to a therapist who is both loved for what she has offered and hated for what she could not put right.

The goodbye letter

A central, organizing strategy in the ending phase involves the therapist writing a goodbye letter to the patient. This is an important feature of cognitive analytic therapy (CAT) (Ryle, 1990, 2004) and we have directly borrowed from this model the idea of including a goodbye letter as part of the DIT protocol. We have done so because it is, in our view, a very helpful intervention that assists the work of ending the therapy and may even be beneficial in preventing relapse (the latter is a hypothesis that requires testing). Unlike CAT, however, the DIT therapist does not write a reformulation letter in the early stages of the treatment—only at the end.

Why a letter? There are a number of reasons why we consider this to be an important adjunct. From a practical point of view a "goodbye letter" provides a helpful way of punctuating the beginning of the ending phase and provides a tangible focus for the joint evaluation of the therapy. In a brief therapy, where the pace and rate of learning for the patient are inevitably faster than in longer-term psychodynamic therapy, the scope for consolidating gains is correspondingly more limited. The letter provides a record of the therapeutic work that the patient can refer to and reconsider once the therapy is over.

For many patients, as Ryle (2004) recognized, the letter is also important because it has the quality of permanence (Hamill et al., 2008). The letter may have symbolic value where the patient's own narrative is characterized by the impermance of his attachments. The letter may thus be said to provide some kind of reassurance at the point of separation—a kind of transitional object that may contribute to the internalization of a benign attachment figure (Ingrassia, 2003). It gives the patient something to take away as a memento of the work and to remind him of the understanding gained if he has later difficult periods, or simply misses the relationship with the therapist.

It is, of course, legitimate and important to raise the possibility that such letters bypass the working through of the pain of separation. Instead of facing loss, patient and therapist could be seen to work together on a letter that somehow avoids the more immediate experience of separation. We would suggest, however, that whilst this possibility needs to be borne in mind and taken up in the transference with the patient where appropriate, in our experience, if the patient's affective experience of ending is addressed directly, as is advocated in DIT, the letter aids the working through of separation rather than avoids it.

Moreover the repeated clinical experience is that these letters provoke strong affects, and are often experienced by the patient as supportive and challenging in equal measure. The letter squarely focuses them on a realistic appraisal of the therapy, what they have gained but also on what it has *not* been possible to achieve, that is, they do not sidestep the reality of disappointment. For the therapist, too, the act of writing the letter can be very powerful and challenging, especially where the work may not have been as successful as she had hoped for.

The discipline of reflecting on the work to arrive at a succinct yet affectively meaningful account of the therapy and its impact on the patient can sometimes alert the therapist to countertransference experiences that she can then take back to the therapy and explore with the patient.

The goodbye letter in practice

In practice we draft a "letter," which functions as both a summary formulation and "progress report," written in terms familiar and accessible to the patient and referring clearly to the IPAF that has been the focus of the work. The letter is a "realistic" account of the work and therefore includes a reference to what has been difficult or challenging for the patient, linking this to a reminder of how the patient managed to overcome these difficulties. Striking the right balance between reminding the patient of his resilience and his ongoing vulnerability is part of the skill in writing these letters, which are typically felt to be challenging and time-consuming by the therapist when they are new to this.

This letter is offered to the patient in session thirteen or fourteen, to give time for the patient to make suggestions, discuss it, and change it. This is intended to be a collaborative process. Even if initiated by us, the final draft should reflect the patient's feedback. Of course, the way the patient relates to this letter is in itself often very interesting. One patient, for example, took the letter away and re-presented it the following week retyped and edited, which left the therapist feeling that the patient had taken it over, leaving her as the abandoned and incompetent one.

The letter should be about a page-and-a-half long, two at most. The language should be jargon-free with an emphasis on putting things as far as possible in the patient's words, or using live examples that have been worked on during the course of therapy and that may have become landmarks of sorts in the work.

When constructing the letter it is helpful to bear in mind the following questions (see Box 10.3):

◆ Does the content capture the IPAF?

◆ Does it communicate clearly and supportively to the patient what change(s) has taken place?

◆ Does it convey a balanced appraisal of the process of the therapy?

- Does it address what it has not been possible to achieve and future goals where relevant?
- Does the tone convey to the patient a sense of the therapist's involvement in the process?

Revisiting the attachment descriptors

In session fourteen or fifteen it is helpful to revisit the attachment statements the patient had rated in session one. The patient is asked to rate himself again on the same statements. Together patient and therapist then reflect on what aspects have changed and what the patient may still wish to change.

It is very unusual to observe significant shifts in these scores because attachment patterns are unlikely to change over such a short period of time. But where it may be possible to note changes is in the patient's more realistic appraisal of what they find difficult or in his wished-for changes in this respect. The questionnaires are thus used primarily as prompts for this kind of evaluative reflection rather than for assessing outcome in any formal sense. It is important to make this clear to the patient who may otherwise be left with the feeling that he or the therapy have failed.

Examples of goodbye letters

Here are some examples of letters. There are some individual variations in style as they have been written by different therapists, but they also share some common characteristics which reflect some of the key principles we outlined earlier (see Box 10.3).

This was the letter Timothy's therapist wrote (see p. 116 for the case study summary):

Dear Timothy,

As our sessions are coming to an end, I have written down my thoughts about the work we have done together. This letter is for you to take away as a reminder of the work and the changes you have made, as well as an acknowledgment of some of the things you may continue to struggle with and work on.

You initially came to your GP wanting help with feelings of depression. At the beginning of your sessions with me, you talked about how

Box 10.3 Guidelines for writing the goodbye letter

The letter should cover the following with an emphasis on the collaborative nature of the work (i.e., the "we-ness" of the experience):

- What has been worked on (i.e., the IPAF)
- What problems/challenges have been encountered
- What has been achieved (i.e., what has been helpful in managing the challenges)
- What remains outstanding

easily and how often you feel like "a loser" in relation to other people whom you expect to treat you badly and to humiliate you in some way. In your description of growing up in your family, I could understand how these feelings about yourself and others may have come to be. During our work together, we discovered how much of an effort you put into trying to resolve this situation and how these things actually might make things worse for you and contribute to your depression.

One of the things we talked about was how, rather than risk being treated badly and feeling like a loser, you keep other people at arm's length (DTA—"don't trust anybody"). You do this by, in a sense, "being on the run" from really being known by other people, and by yourself. We realized how sometimes you do this by being "speedy," sometimes by trying to be the favorite or most special, and sometimes by not being honest with yourself or others about yourself (the "false" Timothy that we got to know a bit). We looked at how this makes you feel, at times, that you don't know who you are. By always being on the run from others, in case they treat you badly or see you as "a loser," you find yourself feeling very lonely and this makes you feel sad.

We also noticed together that sometimes you get yourself into trouble by doing things that appear, at first, to reverse the situation and make someone else into a loser (like the Japanese tourists or the guy in the loading bay at work), and put you in the position of being the one who humiliates someone or treats them badly. What we realized though is that this doesn't actually make you feel any better, at least in the long term. What it does is that it keeps you feeling like a loser because you lose jobs and make enemies. It also stops other people (most of all your family) from getting to know the "real" Timothy.

As the sessions together progressed, you experimented with doing things a bit differently. You tried to be more "real" with others (and we struggled together to allow you to be more "real" with me), to be less "speedy" at work, and to not always have to be the "golden boy." This was not always easy and I know that you are still struggling with allowing the "real" Timothy, who may not always be the "golden boy" or "Jack the lad," but is not a "honeymonster" either, to have a voice. It would not be helpful to think that this is something that will happen quickly or easily. I think that sometimes you believe that you can achieve this by going somewhere else, or leaving without telling anyone where you are going.

I know that you are still struggling with feeling depressed at times and I think that we have to acknowledge that you have started a journey rather than completed it. You have been really courageous though, in making changes in your life outside and in the therapy with me. I hope this letter is useful in highlighting the insights you have gained and that you can use it to help you to continue to allow the "real" Timothy to be more present.

With best wishes

This was the letter Graham's therapist wrote (see p. 176 for the case study summary):

Dear Graham,

As our sessions are coming to an end I have written down my thoughts about the work we have done together. This letter is for you to take away as a reminder of the work and the changes you have made.

You initially came to your GP wanting help with feelings of depression and "melancholia." At the beginning of your sessions with me you were preoccupied with bodily aches and pains and felt "old and fragile." We quickly began to see how your sense of yourself in relation to others was clearly linked to these feelings of depression. You have been able to show me your "wonky" self and how you easily expect to feel criticized, even humiliated, by others, leaving you feeling even more "wonky," irritable, depressed, and inferior. We were able to explore together how you understandably want to protect yourself from this by working hard to keep yourself in a "one up," "special," and superior position. You talked about how your work has played a large part in keeping you in a "special" position and that this had been a motivating force and to a certain extent "kept you going."

As the sessions progressed, however, we have seen how this familiar way of relating has been more limiting, particularly in friendships and more intimate relationships. We have explored your anxiety about getting close to others and a difficulty with asking for and accepting help. You have been worried about someone "taking the whole hand." We have seen clear examples of this, particularly in your relationship with your partner, when she has invited you to be close and you have felt yourself "closing down." You very helpfully have identified your tendency to spoil and sabotage experiences when you feel threatened.

It would be unhelpful to think that these discoveries have been easy and uncomplicated. I have been impressed by your willingness to tackle these difficult issues head on and the many changes you have made in a relatively short space of time. Given your initial anxiety about me being yet another person who would humiliate you or simply see your problems as boring it must have been difficult to let me know what has really been on your mind. It has been helpful to see the relationship with me as a testing ground for other relationships. By doing this you have been able to experience quite a different way of being with somebody. You have been able to open up and show a more vulnerable side of yourself and not immediately feel embarrassed or humiliated. This has allowed you at times to begin to behave differently towards your partner and, in turn, you have experienced her differently. You have identified your greater awareness of these interpersonal dynamics and that you are less ready to "close off" when she invites you to be close or needs your help. You have also been able to stick with the more ordinary "domestic" aspects of a relationship such as going to the supermarket together—which previously you might have reduced to a cliché.

We all need to continue working at our relationships and it would be unrealistic to think that sixteen sessions could have resolved all of the interpersonal difficulties for you. However, you have shown a real capacity for change and we should not underestimate this. I hope this letter is helpful in highlighting this and in motivating you to continue with the valuable work you have started.

With best wishes

This is the letter that Lara's therapist wrote (see p. 137 for the case study summary):

Dear Lara,

As our sessions are coming to an end, I have written down my thoughts about the work we have done together. The letter is for you to take away as a reminder of what you have achieved in the sessions as well as an acknowledgment of some of the things you may still continue to find challenging and may want to continue to work on.

When we first met, you told me that you had been struggling with anxiety and depression most of your life. You mentioned that things had become worse since the birth of your first child. You noticed that you would be okay in relationships for a while but that sooner or later you would hit a "cliff edge" and feel you went "over" and become anxious and depressed. When we looked at this, it seemed to be related to powerful negative feelings you had about yourself especially in relation to other women whom you described jokingly as "the cool kids" to be with. On that note, I was struck by the fact that you viewed yourself as the "geek." You seemed time and time again to see yourself as a failure and different to others, especially other women. When we looked at it more closely we agreed that you felt a constant sense of failure as a "woman" and "mother" and that others could seem harsh and critical of you in this regard or, even more painful, appear so much more "together" and "sorted." This created a lot of anxiety for you in social situations with other mums and eventually you would get down (go over "the cliff"). You also felt this way with women whom you considered "more successful" and "more attractive." To deal with the anxiety you felt you would often push your feelings down and just withdraw or alternatively find a way to show your anger and envy in more civilized ways in veiled criticisms in e-mails or passing comments. Sometimes the emotions would get just so overwhelming that you would just "lose the plot"—as you once described when out socializing one evening.

As we moved on in the sessions, we noticed this pattern happening in several situations in your life, especially with key women you considered to be the ideal. I noticed that in our sessions you would often say "Oh dear, I'm really sorry." We have understood that this was more than likely related to your sense that you may have felt flawed in comparison to me and that you just assumed that I was always right, and moreover the man who was a "model father" with the "perfect kids and family life." This highlighted, even between us, how you often feel flawed and you anticipate that others will be critical of you or humiliate you given the chance.

I know that you still struggle with anxiety and feeling depressed at times. We need to acknowledge that it is unrealistic for sixteen sessions of therapy to completely resolve all ongoing struggles. In a way we have only started a journey rather than completed it. In saying this, I want to really acknowledge and commend you for working hard at looking at painful feelings in our work together.

With best wishes

Working with resistances in the ending phase

When ending stirs a lot of ambivalence it is unsurprising to find that, as the therapy approaches termination, this phase is ripe for acting out. Strictly speaking, acting out refers to the bypassing of a secondary representation of a feeling (e.g. being able to think about a feeling, or even know that it is one as opposed to, for example, construing it as a physical symptom, or boredom, etc.), which is instead expressed indirectly through action. Let us now review some of the most common forms of acting out in the ending phase:

- The *patient misses sessions* (especially the last one). This is one way in which the patient turns what may feel like the passive experience of being left into an active one whereby he is doing the leaving.

- The *patient has nothing to talk about* in the last few sessions. This is often the patient's way of discharging aggression, leaving the therapist feeling impotent and redundant and the one who has to work hard to reach the patient.

- The *patient's symptoms reappear or deteriorate*. Patients often recapitulate old patterns in the termination phase and in so doing express a wish to begin treatment again. Sometimes the deterioration reflects the anxiety generated by the anticipation of leaving the therapist. The return of symptoms may also be used to undermine the therapist, showing her what a bad job she has done as the symptoms have not been "cured."

♦ The *patient displaces hostility onto other figures in his life*. The wish to have a "good" ending can militate against the free expression of ambivalent feelings towards the therapist.

♦ The *patient avoids ending by replacing the therapist* with another therapist or helping figure, thereby reversing the patient's own anticipated experience of being supplanted in the therapist's attentions once the therapy has come to an end. The seamless transition from one therapist to another is another way of denying the pain of separation and loss.

Therapeutic stance in the ending phase

Unlike longer-term psychodynamic therapies that encourage a degree of regression, DIT aims to foster throughout the development of a therapeutic relationship that is more reality-attuned. As we have seen, however, transference distortions will occur and are explored with the patient as the therapy unfolds. One of the tasks of ending involves helping the patient to consolidate a more realistic relationship to the therapist. This is a natural and desirable byproduct of the patient's increasing awareness of his projections.

As the ending approaches we support this more reality-attuned relationship by engaging in a review of the therapy, allying ourselves with the patient's reflecting ego. The experience of two adults taking stock of the work of therapy and thinking about what has changed, and may yet have to change, is a form of collaborative activity that reinforces the patient's adult, more realistic self.

In the final sessions it is helpful to give some realistic appraisal of how the therapy has proceeded and to share with the patient in his achievements without shying away from acknowledging what could not be achieved. Bearing the imperfections of the therapy together is an important part of ending and of helping the patient to develop a realistic relationship with us.

Chapter 11

Frequently Asked Questions

How does DIT differ from interpersonal psychotherapy?

DIT is significantly different from IPT. For a start, IPT is *not* a psychodynamic approach. Both approaches, however, share a clearly identified interpersonal focus and aim to help the patient to address current interpersonal problems. They nevertheless use very different strategies to do so. The IPT therapist achieves this primarily through formulating the patient's symptoms in the context of four predetermined focal areas, each with its specific strategies and goals. By contrast, DIT adopts a very idiographic approach to formulation, selecting a core *unconscious* pattern of interaction that is meaningfully connected to the patient's symptoms/difficulties. Distinctively, whereas DIT deploys the transference relationship as one of the ways of helping the patient work through the identified focus, in IPT the therapist does not work in the transference.

The differences between the two models are clearly reflected in the different competences required to deliver DIT and IPT respectively (see Lemma et al., 2008, 2010).

How does DIT differ from other brief psychodynamic therapies?

DIT explicitly draws on the manuals reviewed as part of the competence framework for the effective delivery of psychodynamic therapy. To this extent we readily expect many colleagues who have developed other brief psychodynamic models to find features of their model reflected in DIT. One of the most interesting outcomes of the work on the competences was to bring to light the significant areas of technical overlap between models drawing on different theoretical traditions in psychoanalysis. All that DIT does is to systematically integrate into one protocol shared psychodynamic principles and techniques, grounded in the extant evidence base, and required to deliver a time-limited intervention with depressed and/or anxious patients. This may be why it appears to be acceptable to therapists trained in a variety of psychodynamic traditions.

Is DIT a supportive psychotherapy?

If all brief psychodynamic models were to be charted on a continuum, ranging from the most expressive/exploratory to the most supportive, then without doubt DIT situates itself at the more supportive end of the spectrum. In this respect it is more explicitly supportive and strengthening of the patient's ego than intensive short-term dynamic psychotherapy (ISTDP), for example, which is more challenging of the patient's defensive structure. However, the supportive components of DIT sit alongside a systematic focus on a segment of the patient's interpersonal functioning, which is typically experienced by the patient as very challenging. The emphasis on helping the patient to try out new ways of managing his relationships, not just on developing insight, is also challenging of the patient's investment in the status quo. DIT therefore does require of the patient some capacity to withstand being challenged in this way. For this reason it would be contraindicated for patients who had no interest in and/or capacity to reflect on some of their own contribution to perpetuating unhelpful dynamics in their relationships.

Is DIT an adaptation of mentalization-based therapy for mood disorders?

We believe that all psychotherapeutic approaches that are helpful to patients more or less explicitly support psychic change through facilitating the patient's capacity to reflect on his states of mind and those of others. The techniques used to this end differ, but the process they facilitate is probably shared. In other words, we see a focus on mentalization as being a core feature of effective interventions with patients across a range of clinical presentations. Maintaining a focus on the patient's mind is core to DIT, which is not quite the same, however, as saying that DIT is just another form of mentalization-based therapy (MBT).

MBT was originally developed for the treatment of borderline patients who typically reveal significant deficits in their capacity to mentalize, hence the assiduous focus on mentalization, which is the hallmark of MBT, along with a range of other interventions targeting the needs of this particular patient group (Bateman and Fonagy, 2006). However, not all depressed or anxious patients share with borderline patients this more characteristic, primary mentalizing deficit, or to the same degree. Of course, we *all* experience failures of mentalization, on a daily basis, and when we feel depressed and/or anxious the capacity to mentalize is undermined to an even greater degree, but these failures are not invariably the *central* deficit in an individual's functioning. This is why within the DIT protocol we explicitly make use of mentalizing techniques to enhance the patient's capacity for reflection when it is weak. However, unlike MBT, DIT is rooted in a psychodynamic approach suited to neurotic patients, with a greater emphasis on the interpretation of transference and of the patient's defensive maneuvers.

Is DIT suitable for patients with personality disorders (PDs)?

DIT has not been developed for use with patients with PD. There is no question in our minds that some of the patients referred with a label of depression and/or anxiety often also present with a host of other difficulties, which reflect an underlying characterological disturbance. This, in turn, undermines the possibility of working to a focus within a time limit. With such patients the protocol would need to be modified not only at the level of its length, but probably also in other respects. This is an empirical question that we have not as yet researched.

We can already see, however, some potential advantages to offering some follow-up or maintenance sessions to those patients who present with a history of chronic depression and/or anxiety. Again this is something that requires further investigation in outcome trials.

How central is working in the transference in DIT?

The simple answer is that it *is* very central, but this requires some qualification because it would not be accurate to say that it is an exclusive or even primary focus. DIT draws on a range of other interventions, such as more supportive interventions, mentalizing interventions, and more sparingly some directive interventions. In DIT the therapist approaches the clinical situation with three main therapeutic priorities in mind, namely (a) to help the patient to explore the IPAF, (b) to help him to reflect on his states of mind, and (c) to make some changes in relation to the problematic relational pattern. The choice of techniques is determined by these priorities, hence the transference is used when and if it supports these strategies, which in practice is often, but not always. It is, however, the case that the DIT therapist *always* uses the transference to understand the patient even if this does not necessarily result in its direct interpretation.

What training do I need to practice DIT?

DIT was explicitly developed to support psychodynamically trained therapists and counselors to hone their existing skills and experience in order to deliver a brief psychodynamic intervention for the treatment of mood disorders. Entry into the training therefore requires a diploma level or equivalent qualification in psychodynamic therapy or counseling followed by a four-day course and two supervised cases, which are audiotaped and rated for adherence to the protocol. This is not a protocol that can be implemented without prior demonstrable competence in working psychodynamically, but it does not require a prior training in intensive (i.e., more than once weekly) psychodynamic therapy.

Does the length of the therapy need to be restricted to sixteen sessions as set out in this protocol?

No. In developing this protocol, we set the number of sessions at sixteen because this was consistent with many other models of brief intervention. We wanted to develop a protocol that would allow us also to test its effectiveness in outcome trials; hence making the length of the treatment comparable to other brief models guided the decision about the number of sessions. Moreover it is our clinical experience that in sixteen sessions much can be achieved with the patient. It is also a reasonable length of time that is acceptable within the confines of delivering psychological therapy in a public health service context.

Given that there is nothing magical about "sixteen," there is nothing inherently problematic about offering a longer or shorter period of time, whilst retaining the overall DIT focus. However, we would guard against simply extending the contract beyond sixteen sessions if this is a way of bypassing the painful reality of ending that has to be faced and processed, and which the patient, and sometimes the therapist too, may be unconsciously avoiding.

Does the DIT therapist work with dreams and unconscious fantasies?

Yes, most definitely. However, as we have emphasized throughout this book, the primary strategy in DIT is to support the working through of the selected IPAF. In other words, dreams and unconscious fantasies may be interpreted if they serve the function of illustrating to the patient the activation of the IPAF in his current life and interpersonal context.

Does the DIT therapist use the countertransference as the basis for intervening?

Yes. Using the countertransference to inform the therapist's understanding of what is transpiring between herself and the patient is central to DIT. Without consideration of the impact the patient has on the therapist we cannot see how therapists could arrive at a comprehensive understanding of the patient or how they can effectively manage difficulties in the therapeutic relationship.

Does DIT focus on the patient's past?

Yes and no. DIT is underpinned by an understanding of developmental theory, which contextualizes the patient's current functioning in light of developmental models of self-in-relation-to-an-other, which have been internalized on the basis of early experience with significant attachment figures. Whilst such an understanding of the early origins of our internalized object relationships is important, the focus of the therapist's efforts is to help the patient understand the way in which the pattern itself is active in his *current* life and relationships.

The focus in DIT on the activation in the present of internalized object relationships is consistent with most contemporary psychodynamic models, where reconstruction of the past is no longer regarded as the primary intervention leading to psychic change. Having said this, given DIT's brevity and the importance of formulation within this protocol, there is value in helping the patient to contextualize his difficulties with reference to significant experiences in his life, which may feel especially salient for him, or that may have been neglected in an unhelpful way. The *formulation* in DIT therefore draws on an understanding of the early origins of the problems to provide the patient with a narrative that will orientate him to the task in hand, which is nevertheless focused on working on the present.

What should I expect if I choose to train in DIT?

The first thing to say is that it is always harder (not least on one's narcissism!) to learn an adaptation of an already acquired model. This is partly because learning to deliver an adaptation, such as DIT, will expose you to familiar ideas and techniques (and hence ones that you will most likely feel competent in), but which are nevertheless integrated in ways that will feel more or less unfamiliar, and hence that may leave you feeling somehow wrong-footed and incompetent. It may possibly also feel in conflict with a training superego that proscribes some of the techniques that are actively encouraged in this protocol.

In our experience, the steepest learning curve is in the requirement to explicitly formulating a focus and working assiduously to this focus. This involves tolerating what often feels like "ignoring" fascinating aspects of the patient's varied and complex mental life. This is often felt to be more challenging even than integrating outcome monitoring in every session.

Appendix 1

DIT Competences

Brief dynamic interpersonal therapy (DIT) for depression

This section describes the knowledge and skills required to carry out DIT.

It is not a "stand-alone" description of technique, and should be read as part of the psychoanalytic/psychodynamic competence framework (see www.ucl.ac.uk/CORE).

Effective delivery of this approach depends on the integration of this competence list with the knowledge and skills set out in the other domains of the psychoanalytic/psychodynamic competence framework.

Knowledge
General

An ability to draw on knowledge of the psychological and interpersonal difficulties experienced by patients with a diagnosis of depression

Knowledge of the developmental model underpinning the understanding of depression

An ability to draw on knowledge that DIT is grounded in attachment theory (including models of mentalization), object-relations theory, and interpersonal psychoanalysis

An ability to draw on knowledge of attachment-based and object-relational models of depression

Knowledge of the aims and focus of treatment

An ability to draw on knowledge that DIT aims to help the patient:

> understand the connection between his presenting symptoms and significant difficulties in his relationships, by working with him to identify a core, unconscious, repetitive pattern of relating (and making this the focus of the therapy)

> develop a capacity to mentalize

An ability to draw on knowledge that the primary aim of DIT is to enhance the patient's interpersonal functioning and his capacity to think about and relate changes in his mood to mental states (conscious and nonconscious)

An ability to draw on knowledge that DIT systematically focuses on:

> a circumscribed IPAF that is linked with the onset and/or maintenance of symptoms

> the patient's state of mind, rather than his behavior

> the patient's experience in the here and now of the session or recent past, rather than the interpretation of distal events

Knowledge of the treatment strategy

An ability to draw on knowledge that the three main phases of the treatment have distinct aims:

> an *initial* phase that aims to assess the quality and patterning of relationships, past and present, as the basis for identifying a dominant, recurring, unconscious IPAF that will become the focus of the therapy

> a *middle* phase that focuses on helping the patient to elaborate and work on the IPAF

> an *ending* phase that focuses on helping the patient to reflect on the affective experience of ending and so prepare for ending and plan for the future

An ability to draw on knowledge that DIT makes active use of the patient–therapist relationship to explore the IPAF

An ability to draw on knowledge that DIT makes use of expressive, supportive, and directive techniques to support the aims of the treatment

Interventions
Therapeutic stance

An ability to establish and maintain an involved, empathic relationship with the patient

An ability to establish and sustain an active, collaborative stance

An ability to adopt a "not-knowing," curious stance when exploring the patient's mental states, to communicate a genuine attempt to find out about his mental experience

Ability to assess the severity of the patient's depression

An ability to assess the patient's overall functioning to arrive at a diagnosis of depression

An ability to assess level of risk

An ability to involve relevant professional networks to support the therapy where appropriate

Ability to assess the quality and patterning of the patient's current and past interpersonal functioning and formulate a focus

An ability to generate, clarify, and elaborate narratives about relationships

An ability to draw the patient's attention to repetitive patterns in his relationships

An ability to identify one dominant repetitive interpersonal pattern that is connected to the onset/maintenance of the depression and that will become the focus of the therapy (IPAF)

An ability actively to reflect on, and make use of, the transference relationship, and the therapist's countertransfence, to arrive at the formulation of the IPAF

Ability to engage the patient in DIT

An ability to communicate with the patient in a direct, transparent manner that invites him to provide feedback on the formulation and process of therapy:

an ability to respond to requests by the patient for clarification in a direct and clear manner that models a self-reflective stance that is open to correction

An ability to offer a "trial interpretation" in order to:

make use of the patient's response to the interpretation in order to elaborate the evolving formulation

assess the patient's capacity to make use of such interventions

An ability to engage the patient in formulating the focus of the work by:

tentatively sharing an understanding of how his presenting symptoms/problems may be connected with unconscious feelings and interpersonal conflicts

actively soliciting the patient's response to the formulation and engaging reflection on his emotional reaction to it

modifying the formulation in line with new understanding developed with the patient

An ability to introduce the patient to the rationale and aims of DIT through the use of "live" material in the session (e.g. by drawing the patient's attention to recurring interpersonal dynamics as he describes himself and his relationships)

an ability to personalize the introduction of the model by linking it to the patient's own history, current symptoms, and interpersonal experiences

Ability to help the patient identify his aims for the therapy

An ability to identify and agree with the patient therapeutic goals that are meaningfully connected with the agreed IPAF

An ability to help the patient to be realistic about what can be achieved within a brief time frame:

an ability to respond to any feelings the patient has about areas it may not be possible to work on

Ability to work to the agreed focus

An ability to elicit INs and to track the agreed IPAF as it emerges in the narrative(s) as the basis for any interpretation

An ability to maintain a focus on *current* significant relationships that demonstrate the activation of the IPAF and its relationship to depression:

an ability to take a stance of curiosity about interpersonal scenarios (e.g. asking questions and for clarifications as necessary, to bring into focus an interpersonal exchange so as to highlight a salient repetitive pattern)

An ability to maintain a focus on the agreed IPAF by:

identifying areas of difficulty in the patient's relationships that relate to the IPAF

understanding the patient's characteristic ways of managing areas of difficulty in his relationships and to point out the "cost" of these strategies

inviting reflection on the unconscious assumptions behind feelings and thoughts when in a relationship in order to highlight the way these assumptions perpetuate or exacerbate interpersonal difficulties

drawing the patient's attention to his affective state in the session

attending to the therapeutic relationship in order to draw the patient's attention to moments when the relationship between therapist and patient reflects the activation of the agreed IPAF

helping the patient practice the skill of recognizing internal states (feelings and thoughts) as they relate to the IPAF

Ability to focus the content of interventions

An ability to focus on the patient's mind, not on his behavior:

an ability to follow shifts and changes in the patient's understanding of his own and others' thoughts and feelings

An ability to focus on the patient's affects (primarily in relation to the here and now of the session and his current circumstances)

An ability to focus on current relationships, including the relationship with the therapist

Ability to work collaboratively with the patient towards an understanding of the transference experience

An ability to help the patient to be curious about what is happening in the therapeutic relationship

An ability to identify and respond to enactments/ruptures in the therapeutic relationship:

an ability to respond nondefensively to the patient's experience of the therapist

an ability to use clarification and elaboration to elicit a detailed picture of what has transpired between the patient and therapist

an ability to monitor countertransference and to work to regain a reflective stance after an enactment

an ability to acknowledge and explore openly with the patient any enactments on the part of the therapist

an ability to communicate the therapist's perspective about the impasse or rupture

An ability to monitor and engage with the patient's response to an interpretation

Ability to support the patient's mentalizing stance in relation to the IPAF

An ability to use clarification and elaboration to gather a detailed picture of the feelings associated with a specific behavioral sequence related to the IPAF

An ability to help the patient make connections between actions and feelings

An ability to help the patient develop curiosity about his motivations

An ability for the therapist to share her perspective so as to help the patient to consider an alternative experience of the same event

An ability to help the patient shift the focus from nonmentalizing interaction with the therapist towards an exploration of current feelings and thoughts (as manifested in the patient–therapist interaction, or in recent experiences outside the therapy room)

Ability to encourage interpersonal change

An ability to balance helping the patient to explore the IPAF and supporting him to make use of his understanding of the IPAF to change current relationship patterns that are linked with the onset and/or maintenance of depression

An ability to monitor and respond to the patient's experience of the therapist's more active stance

Ability to integrate routine outcome monitoring into the therapeutic process

An ability to engage the patient in reflecting on his responses to the questionnaires:

an ability to respond to the patient's use of the questionnaires in the context of the evolving transference relationship

An ability to use and interpret weekly questionnaire data in order to track progress, and to guide any changes to the intervention indicated by these data (e.g. in response to evidence of a deterioration in levels of depression)

Ability to explore the unconscious and affective experience of ending

An ability to assess the patient's sensitivity to separation so as to ensure that the meaning of the ending is worked on from the outset

An ability systematically to draw attention to, and explore, the patient's feelings, unconscious fantasies, and anxieties about the ending of therapy

An ability to recognize and respond to indications of regression near the end of treatment (e.g. a symptomatic deterioration) by linking this with the feelings and fantasies associated with endings

An ability to help the patient to review the therapy as a whole (e.g. whether he has achieved his aims):

an ability to help the patient express disappointment where appropriate

an ability to respond nondefensively to the patient's feedback about the therapy

An ability to compose a "goodbye" letter which reviews the original agreed formulation and progress made in working on the issues identified at the start of therapy:

an ability to engage the patient in responding to and refining the letter

Patient Information Leaflet

Dynamic interpersonal therapy (DIT) for depression and anxiety

What is DIT?

DIT is a time-limited (sixteen sessions) psychodynamic therapy that can help people with emotional and relationship problems. It has been specifically developed for the treatment of depression and anxiety.

One of the main ideas in psychodynamic therapy is that when something is very painful we can find ourselves trying to ignore it (it's a bit like the saying "out of sight, out of mind"). Most of the time we know when we're doing this, but sometimes we can bury something so successfully that we lose sight of it completely. This is why difficult experiences in the past can continue to affect the way we feel and behave in the present. DIT provides people with a safe place to talk openly about how they feel and to understand what might be causing their difficulties.

An example shows how this might work. Someone who was repeatedly rejected by their parents may stop themselves thinking about how painful this is. As an adult they might become depressed, withdraw from relationships, feeling that it is safer to be alone and not having to depend on anyone. Although not getting close to anyone helps them to feel safer, they might also feel lonely and get depressed as a result.

How would a DIT therapist help such a person? By helping them to talk freely about themselves it might become clear that whenever someone tries to get to know them, they fear the worst and push them away, just to make sure that no-one ever gets close enough to hurt or disappoint them again. In the course of day-to-day life people don't necessarily notice how they are behaving or responding to others because this becomes second nature—"the way things are." By drawing their attention to this *pattern*, therapy would help them to understand themselves better and change the way they respond.

What does therapy involve?

Everyone's therapy will be a bit different, but we have tried to describe some of the important things that a good therapist will do and what they will help you focus on.

Starting off

All therapists should be able to help you feel respected and comfortable. Many people find it difficult to talk about their problems with someone they do not know, and it is important that your therapist can make you feel that they are to be trusted, and can help you manage if you talk about things that upset you or about which you feel embarrassed.

Talking openly about yourself for the first time to a new person can feel difficult and you may be worried about what your therapist thinks about you. Your therapist will be interested in how you experience them and will help you to make sense of any worries you may have about starting therapy. They should give you the feeling that they know that starting therapy can be difficult and that they understand what life is like for you.

Getting a picture of what you need (assessment)

Your therapist will need to get as good a picture as they can of what you are finding difficult in your life and how this is affecting you and people close to you. They will ask some questions, but they should also make it clear that you only need to give as much information as you feel comfortable with. Many people find that, as therapy gets going, they are able to talk more openly, and in the early stages you shouldn't find yourself under pressure to say more than you want.

Although your therapist will need to gather some basic information about you and your life, and your relationships in particular, some of the time they will wait for you to talk. This is because they are interested in hearing about what is on your mind rather than asking you lots of questions. Sometimes your therapist may remain silent, waiting for you to speak. This may well feel a bit uncomfortable—for example, you may feel unsure what to say. However, if this gets too uncomfortable, your therapist will help you talk.

At the start of therapy your therapist will ask you to complete some questionnaires. These will give them a better idea of the sorts of problems you have (by asking about the sort of difficulties you have), as well as how badly these affect you (by asking how much each problem affects you). Your therapist will discuss the results of these questionnaires with you. They will ask you to complete the questionnaires again every session because this helps you and your therapist see what progress you are making. This is very useful, because not everyone makes progress at the same rate. If the questionnaires show that you are not benefiting from therapy, it gives you and your therapist a chance to think about why this might be.

Explaining how DIT might work for you

Early on, your therapist should explain how DIT works, and help you to think through how the approach makes sense of what you're finding difficult in your life. The experience of the assessment should also give you an idea of how the therapy works, what is expected of you, and what you can expect of the therapist. The main thing is that the therapist needs to help you see the ways in which ideas from DIT could be relevant to you and what you want help with. That does not mean you need to be 100 percent convinced at this stage—it's more that the idea of DIT needs to make some sense to you if you are going to get the best out of it.

Sharing ideas about what you want to achieve

When your therapist has enough information they will begin thinking with you about what it would be most helpful for you to focus on over the sixteen sessions. This is also an opportunity to agree with your therapist about what you want out of the therapy.

Length and frequency of treatment

Your therapist will talk with you about the fixed number of sessions you can expect to have. This will typically be sixteen sessions. The therapy usually takes place once a week. Your therapist will discuss with you any planned breaks and what happens if you cancel sessions.

What can you expect of your therapist

Your therapist is responsible for ensuring that your meetings take place at a regular time, in a setting where you can be sure of confidentiality. Wherever possible they should let you know if they expect to be away or need to change the time of your therapy. Sometimes people find breaks from the therapy hard to manage. When this happens your therapist should discuss this with you and help you to understand why this may feel particularly difficult.

Ending the therapy

Many patients find that ending the therapy is difficult. This is because the relationship that develops between you and your therapist can become quite important. Ending therapy can feel like a big loss and you are likely to experience a range of feelings about it. Your therapist will know and understand this and you should expect them to help you to explore your feelings, including any worries you might have about how you will cope in the future. They should help you think about how you would manage if things became difficult again. After all, the aim of DIT isn't to remove your problems—everyone has problems that they need to deal with. The hope is that you will have learned how to manage better, and so avoid problems becoming major difficulties again.

Some important features of psychodynamic therapy

1. One important feature of DIT is that it uses what happens in the relationship between therapist and patient to help you think about the problems in your life. An example would help to clarify what we mean by this. Remember the person we described at the start of this leaflet, who worries about getting rejected by people. As they settle into therapy they might start to worry that the therapist will reject them too—for example, they could become convinced that the therapist wasn't really interested in them. The therapist might comment on their concern because this would provide a clear illustration of where things go wrong in the patient's relationships. By discussing the similarity between the worries they have about the therapist and

the worries they have in general, the patient would start to get a better picture of what happens to them in relationships. In practice this means that the therapist will often draw your attention to what you are currently feeling in the session. The idea is that, by exploring the relationship between you and your therapist, you can get a better understanding of what is troubling you.

2. As discussed earlier, you may find that your therapist is a bit more "silent" than you might be used to. For example, at the beginning of each session your therapist will greet you and will ask you to fill in some questionnaires, but beyond this may not ask questions. Instead they will wait to hear from you about what is on your mind. This is not because they are being "unfriendly," but because they want you to have some space to work out what is on your mind. This can take a while to get used to, but your therapist will know how hard it can be and should help if you find this particularly difficult.

3. Another feature of DIT is that the therapist won't always answer your questions directly. Sometimes they may be interested in what lies behind your questions. For example, someone who is very worried about starting therapy may not feel able to say this straightforwardly. Instead they may ask lots and lots of questions about what therapy involves. Rather than answering all of these directly, the therapist may notice that behind the questions is a worry about beginning therapy. Helping the patient talk about this, rather than answering all the questions, is probably a more helpful way forward.

Appendix 3

DIT Rating Form

DIT Session Rating Form

Therapist: .... **Session #:** ....

Client ID: .... **Rater:** ....

Instructions: Using the scale provided below, please rate how characteristic each statement was of the therapy session. For each item, please write the scale rating number on the blank line provided.

Scale:

0		1	2		3	4		5	6
Not at all characteristic			Somewhat characteristic			Characteristic			Highly characteristic

1. The therapist works collaboratively with the patient to formulate and agree an IPAF and related goals _____ (*initial sessions only*)

2. The therapist encourages the exploration of feelings _____

3. The therapist focuses on the patient's mind rather than his behavior (links interpersonal processes with patient's mental states) _____

4. The therapist focuses discussion on the agreed IPAF _____

5. The therapist focuses on the exploration of interpersonal events _____

6. The therapist helps the patient to discover what he *currently* feels and how this relates to current and past interpersonal experiences _____

7. The therapist helps the patient to make connections between symptoms and interpersonal events _____

8. The therapist maintains an active, supportive stance to encourage the patient to try out new ways of resolving his interpersonal difficulties in between sessions _____

9. The therapist gives explicit advice or direct suggestions to the patient _____

10. The therapist actively initiates the topics of discussion and therapeutic activities _____

11. The therapist links the patient's current feelings or perceptions to experiences of the past _____

12. The therapist focuses attention on similarities among the patient's relationships repeated over time, settings, or people _____

13. The therapist focuses discussion on the patient's irrational or illogical belief systems _____

14. The therapist focuses discussion on the relationship between the therapist and patient in order to further the exploration of the IPAF _____

15. The therapist encourages the patient to experience and express feelings in the session _____

16. The therapist addresses the patient's avoidance of important topics and shifts in mood _____

17. The therapist explains the rationale behind her technique or approach to treatment _____

18. The therapist suggests alternative ways to understand experiences or events not previously recognized by the patient _____

19. The therapist identifies recurrent patterns in the patient's actions, feelings, and experiences _____

20. The therapist provides the patient with information and facts about his current symptoms, disorder, or treatment _____

21. The therapist allows the patient to initiate the discussion of significant issues, events, and experiences _____

22. The therapist teaches the patient specific techniques for coping with symptoms _____

23. The therapist encourages discussion of the patient's wishes, fantasies, dreams, or early childhood memories (positive or negative) _____

24. The therapist interacts with the patient in a didactic manner _____

Ending phase sessions only

25. The therapist facilitates the expression of the patient's anxieties and fantasies about ending _____

26. The therapist helps the patient to review work that has been accomplished _____

27. The therapist engages the patient in anticipating future difficulties/areas of vulnerability _____

References

Abbass, A., Hancock, J., Henderson, J., & Kisely, S. (2007). Short-term psychodynamic psychotherapies for common mental disorders (Review). *Cochrane Database of Systematic Reviews 2006*, Issue 4. Art. No.: CD004687. DOI: 004610001002/14651858.CD14004687.pub14651853.

Abbass, A., Sheldon, A., Gyra, J., & Kalpin, A. (2008). Intensive short-term dynamic psychotherapy for DSM IV personality disorders. A randomized controlled trial and Anger. *J Nervous and Mental Disease, 196*, 1–6.

Abramson, L. Y., Seligman, M. E. P. and Teasdale, J. D. (1978). Learned helplessness in humans: critique and reformulation. *Journal of Abnormal Psychology, 87*, 49–74.

Akhtar, S. (1992). *Broken Structures: Sever Personality Disorders and Their Treatment*. Northvale, New Jersey: Jason Aronson.

Allen, J., Fonagy, P. and Bateman, A. (2008). *Mentalizing in Clinical Practice*. Washington, DC: American Psychiatric Press.

American Psychiatric Association. (1980). *Diagnostic and Statistical Manual of Mental Disorders 3rd edn, DSM-III*. Washington, DC: American Psychiatric Press.

Angst, J. and Dobler-Mikola, A. (1985). The Zurich Study. VI. A continuum from depression to anxiety disorders? *European Archives of Psychiatry and Neurological Science, 235*, 179–86.

Bacal, H. (1990). Does an object relations theory exist in self psychology? *Psychoanalytical Inquiry, 10*, 197–220.

Bachar, E., Latzer, Y., Kreitler, S. and Berry, E. M. (1999). Empirical comparison of two psychological therapies. Self psychology and cognitive orientation in the treatment of anorexia and bulimia. *Journal of Psychotherapy Practice and Research, 8*(2), 115–28.

Bakermans-Kranenburg, M. J., Van Ijzendoorn, M. H., Mesman, J., Alink, L. R. and Juffer, F. (2008). Effects of an attachment-based intervention on daily cortisol moderated by dopamine receptor D4: a randomized control trial on 1- to 3-year-olds screened for externalizing behavior. *Development and Psychopathology, 20*(3), 805–20.

Baldwin, S. A., Wampold, B. E. and Imel, Z. E. (2007). Untangling the alliance-outcome correlation: exploring the relative importance of therapist and patient variability in the alliance. *Journal of Consulting and Clinical Psychology, 75*(6), 842–52.

Balint, M. (1937). Early developmental states of the ego, primary object of love *Primary love and psycho-analytic technique* (pp. 90–108). London: Tavistock, 1968.

Balint, M. (1968). *The basic fault*. London: Tavistock.

Barry, R. A., Kochanska, G. and Philibert, R. A. (2008). G x E interaction in the organization of attachment: mothers' responsiveness as a moderator of children's genotypes. *Journal of Child Psychology and Psychiatry, 49*(12), 1313–20.

Bartholomew, K. and Horowitz, L. M. (1991). Attachment styles among young adults: a test of a four-category model. *Journal of Personality and Social Psychology, 61*, 226–44.

Bateman, A. W. and Fonagy, P. (1999). The effectiveness of partial hospitalization in the treatment of borderline personality disorder—a randomised controlled trial. *American Journal of Psychiatry, 156*, 1563–9.

Bateman, A. W. and Fonagy, P. (2006). *Mentalization-based Treatment for Borderline Personality Disorder: A Practical Guide*. Oxford: Oxford University Press.

Bateman, A. W. and Fonagy, P. (2008). 8-year follow-up of patients treated for borderline personality disorder—mentalization-based treatment versus treatment as usual. *American Journal of Psychiatry, 165*(5), 631–8.

Bateman, A., Brown, D. and Pedder, J. (2000). *Introduction to Psychotherapy: An Outline of Psychodynamic Principles and Practice*, 3rd edn. London: Routledge.

Beck, A. T. and Bhar, S. S. (2009). Analyzing effectiveness of long-term psychodynamic psychotherapy. *Journal of the American Medical Association, 301*(9), 931; author reply 932–33.

Beck, A. T., Rush, J., Shaw, B. and Emery, G. (1979). *Cognitive Therapy of Depression*. New York: Guilford.

Bifulco, A., Moran, P. M., Ball, C. and Bernazzani, O. (2002a). Adult attachment style. I: Its relationship to clinical depression. *Social Psychiatry and Psychiatric Epidemiology, 37*, 50–9.

Bifulco, A., Moran, P. M., Ball, C. and Lillie, A. (2002b). Adult attachment style. II: Its relationship to psychosocial depressive-vulnerability. *Social Psychiatry and Psychiatric Epidemiology, 37*, 60–7.

Binder, J. (2004). *Key Competences in Brief Psychodynamic Therapy: Clinical Practice Beyond the Manual*. London: The Guilford Press.

Blackmore, M., Erwin, B. A., Heimberg, R. G., Magee, L., and Fresco, D. M. (2009). Social anxiety disorder and specific phobias. In: Gelder, M. G., Lopez-Ibor, J. J., Andreason, N. C., Geddes, J. (eds.). *New Oxford textbook of psychiatry*. 2nd ed. Oxford: Oxford University Press.

Blatt, S. J. (2008). *Polarities of Experience: Relatedness and Self Definition in Personality Development, Psychopathology, and the Therapeutic Process*. Washington, DC: American Psychological Association.

Blatt, S. J. and Luyten, P. (2009). A structural-developmental psychodynamic approach to psychopathology: two polarities of experience across the life span. *Development and Psychopathology, 21*(3), 793–814.

Blatt, S. J., Zuroff, D. C., Hawley, L. L. and Auerbach, J. S. (2010). Predictors of sustained therapeutic change. *Psychotherapy Research, 20*(1), 37–54.

Bögels, S. M., Wijts, P. and Sallaerts, S. (2003). Analytic psychotherapy versus cognitive-behavioral therapy for social phobia. Paper presented at the *EABCT Congress*, Prague.

Bollas, C. (1996). Figures and their function: The oedipal structure of psychoanalysis. *Psychoanalytic Quarterly, 65*, 1–20.

Bolognini, S. (2006). The profession of ferryman: considerations on the analyst's internal attitude in consultation and referral. In B. Reith, S. Lagerlof, P. Crick, M. Moller, and E. Skale (eds), *Initiating Psychoanalysis*. London: Routledge.

Book, H. (1998). *How to Practice Brief Psychodynamic Psychotherapy: The CCRT Method*. Washington, DC: American Psychiatric Association.

Bowlby, J. (1969). *Attachment and Loss, Vol. 1: Attachment*. London: Hogarth Press and the Institute of Psycho-Analysis.

Bowlby, J. (1973). *Attachment and Loss, Vol. 2: Separation: Anxiety and Anger*. London: Hogarth Press and Institute of Psycho-Analysis.

Bowlby, J. (1980). *Attachment and Loss, Vol. 3: Loss: Sadness and Depression*. London: Hogarth Press and Institute of Psycho-Analysis.

Bravesmith, A. (2010). CAN WE BE BRIEF? *British Journal of Psychotherapy, 26*, 274–90. doi:10.1111/j.1752-0118.2010.01186.

Brent, D., Emslie, G., Clarke, G., Wagner, K. D., Asarnow, J. R., Keller, M. et al. (2008). Switching to another SSRI or to venlafaxine with or without cognitive behavioral therapy for adolescents with SSRI-resistant depression: the TORDIA randomized controlled trial. *Journal of the American Medical Association, 299*(8), 901–13.

Bretherton, I. (1985). Attachment theory: Retrospect and prospect. *Monographs of the Society for Research in Child Development, 50*(1–2), 3–35.

Bretherton, K. and Munholland, K. A. (1999). Internal working models in attachment relationships: A construct revisited. In J. Cassidy & P. R. Shaver (eds.), *Handbook of Attachment: Theory, Research and Clinical Applications*, (pp. 89–114). New York: Guilford Press.

Briggs, S., Lemma, A. and Crouch, W. (eds) (2008). *Relating to Self-harm and Suicide: Psychoanalytic Perspectives on Practice, Theory and Prevention*. London: Routledge.

Britton, R. (2003). *Sex, Death and the Superego*. London: Karnac.

Brown, G. W. and Harris, T. O. (1978). *Social Origins of Depression: A Study of Psychiatric Disorders in Women*. London: Tavistock.

Brown, G. W. and Harris, T. O. (1989). *Life Events and Illness*. London: Unwin Hyman.

Busch, F. and Milrod, B. (2010). The ongoing struggle for psychoanalytic research: some steps forward. *Psychoanalytic Psychotherapy, 24*(4), 306–14.

Busch, F., Milrod, B. and Sandberg, L. (2009). A study demonstrating the efficacy of psychoanalytic psychotherapy for panic disorder: implications for psycho-analytic research, theroy and practice. *Journal of the American Psychoanalytic Association, 57*, 1131–48.

Calef, V., & Weinshel, E. M. (1980). The Analyst as the Conscience of the Analysis. *Int. Rev. Psycho-Anal., 7*, 279–290.

Carrig, M. M., Kolden, G. G. and Strauman, T. J. (2009). Using functional magnetic resonance imaging in psychotherapy research: A brief introduction to concepts, methods, and task selection. *Psychotherapy Research, 19*(4–5), 409–17.

Caspi, A., Sugden, K., Moffitt, T. E., Taylor, A., Craig, I. W., Harrington, H. et al. (2003). Influence of life stress on depression: moderation by a polymorphism in the 5-HTT gene. *Science, 301*(5631), 386–9.

Chorpita, B. F., & Barlow, D. H. (1998). The development of anxiety: the role of control in the early environment. *Psychol Bull, 124*(1), 3–21.

Cischetti, D. (1990). The organization and coherence of socioemotional, congni-tive, and representational development: Illustrations through a developmental psychopathology perspective on Down syndrome and child maltreatment. In R. Thompson (ed.), *Socioemotional development. Nebraska symposium on motivation* (pp. 259–79). Lincoln: University of Nebraska Press.

Clark, D. M., & Wells, A. (1995). A cognitive model of social phobia. In. R. G. Heimberg, M. R. Liebowitz, D. A. Hope, & F. R. Schneier (Eds.), Social phobia: Diagnosis, assessment, and treatment (pp. 41–68). Guilford Press: New York.

Clarkin, J., Levy, K. N., Lenzenweger, M. F. and Kernberg, O. F. (2007). Evaluating three treatments for borderline personality disorder: a multiwave study. *American Journal of Psychiatry, 164*, 922–8.

Cloitre, M., Chase Stovall-McClough, K., Miranda, R. and Chemtob, C. M. (2004). Therapeutic alliance, negative mood regulation, and treatment outcome in child abuse-related posttraumatic stress disorder. *Journal of Consulting and Clinical Psychology, 72*(3), 411–16.

Cohen, J. (1962). The statistical power of abnormal-social psychological research: a review. *Journal of Abnormal and Social Psychology, 65*, 145–53.

Conradi, H. J. and de Jonge, P. (2009). Recurrent depression and the role of adult attachment: a prospective and a retrospective study. *Journal of Affective Disorders, 116*(1–2), 93–9.

Crits-Christoph, P., Connolly Gibbons, M. B., Narducci, J., Schamberger, M., & Gallop, R. (2005). Interpersonal problems and the outcome of interpersonally oriented psychodynamic treatment of GAD. Psychotherapy: Theory, Research, Practice, Training, *42*, 211–24.

Crittenden, P. M. (1990). Internal representational models of attachment relationships. *Infant Mental Health Journal, 11*, 259–77.

Crittenden, P. M. (1994). Peering into the black box: An exploratory treatise on the development of self in young children. In D. Cicchetti & S. L. Toth (Eds.), *Disorders and dysfunctions of the self. Rochester Symposium on Developmental Psychopatholocy, Vol. 5* (pp. 79–148). Rochester, NY: University of Rochester Press.

Cuijpers, P., van Straten, A., van Oppen, P. and Andersson, G. (2008). Are psychological and pharmacologic interventions equally effective in the treatment of adult depressive disorders? A meta-analysis of comparative studies. *Journal of Clinical Psychiatry, 69*(11), 1675–85; quiz 839–41.

Dare, C., Eisler, I., Russell, G., Treasure, J. and Dodge, L. (2001). Psychological therapies for adults with anorexia nervosa: randomised controlled trial of out-patient treatments. *British Journal of Psychiatry, 178*, 216–21.

de Maat, S., de Jonghe, F., Schoevers, R. and Dekker, J. (2009). The effectiveness of long-term psychoanalytic therapy: a systematic review of empirical studies. *Harvard Review of Psychiatry, 17*(1), 1–23.

Dekker, J. J. M., Koelen, J. A., Van, H. L., Schoevers, R. A., Peen, J., Hendriksen, M., et al. (2008). Speed of action: The relative efficacy of short-term psychodynamic supportive psychotherapy and pharmacotherapy in the first 8 weeks of a treatment algorithm for depression. *Journal of Affective disorders, 109*, 183–8.

Dolan, P., Lee, H. J., King, D. and Metcalpe, R. (2009). How does NICE value health? *British Medical Journal, 339*, 371–3.

Driessen, E., Cuijpers, P., de Maat, S., Abbass, A., de Jonghe, F., & Dekker, J. (2010). The efficacy of short-term psychodynamic psychotherapy for depression: A meta-analysis. *Clin Psych Rev, 30*, 25–36.

Durham, R. C., Murphy, T., Allan, T., Richard, K., Treliving, L. R., & Fenton, G. W. (1994). Cognitive therapy, analytic psychotherapy and anxiety management training for generalized anxiety disorder. British Journal of Psychiatry, *165*, 315–23.

Dwal, S., & Tweedie, R. (2000). Trimm and fill: A simple funnel-plot-based method of testing and adjusting for publication bias in meta-analysis. *Biometrics, 56*, 455–463.

Eaton, W., Shao, H., Nesdadt, G., Lee, B., Bienvenu, O. and Zandi, P. (2008) Population-based study of first onset and chronicity in major depressive disorder. *Archives of General Psychiatry, 65*, 513–20.

Eisenberger, N. I., Lieberman, M. D. and Williams, K. D. (2003). Does rejection hurt? An fMRI study of social exclusion. *Science, 302*(5643), 290–92.

Engel, G. L. and Schmale, A. H. Jr. (1967). Psychoanalytic theory of somatic disorder—conversion, specificity, and the disease onset situation. *Journal of the American Psychoanalysis Association, 15*, 344–65.

Etchegoyen, R. H. (1999). *Fundamentals of Psychoanalytic Technique*, revised edn. London: Karnac Books.

Eysenck, H. J. (1952). The effects of psychotherapy: an evaluation. *Journal of Consulting Psychology, 16*, 319–24.

Fairbairn, W. R. D. (1952). *An Object-Relations Theory of the Personality.* New York: Basic Books, 1954.

Fischer-Kern, M., Tmej, A., Kapusta, N. D., Naderer, A., Leithner-Dziubas, K., Löffler-Stastka, H. et al. (2008). Mentalisierungsfähigkeit bei depressiven Patientinnen: Eine Pilotstudie. *Zeitschrift für Psychosomatische Medizin und Psychotherapie, 54,* 368–80.

Fonagy, I. and Fonagy, P. (1995). Communication with pretend actions in language, literature and psychoanalysis. *Psychoanalysis and Contemporary Thought, 18,* 363–418.

Fonagy, P. (1999). Achieving evidence-based psychotherapy practice: a psychodynamic perspective on the general acceptance of treatment manuals. *Clinical Psychology: Science and Practice, 6,* 442–44.

Fonagy, P. (2001). *Attachment Theory in Psychoanalysis.* New York: Other Press.

Fonagy, P. (2010). The changing shape of clinical practice: driven by science or pragmatics? *Psychoanalytic Psychotherapy, 24*(1), 22–43.

Fonagy, P. and Higgitt, A. (2009). *SSRIs: should they be the first line treatment for pediatric depression or should they be banned? A systematic review of not so systematic reviews of the SSRI controversy.* Unpublished manuscript.

Fonagy, P. and Target, M. (2000). Playing with reality III: the persistence of dual psychic reality in borderline patients. *International Journal of Psychoanalysis, 81*(5), 853–74.

Fonagy, P. and Target, M. (2003). *Psychoanalytic Theories: Perspectives from Developmental Psychopathology.* London: Whurr.

Fonagy, P., Dergely, G., Jurist, E. and Target, M. (2004). *Affect Regulation, Mentalization and the Development of the Self.* London: Karnac Books.

Fonagy, P., Leigh, T., Steele, M., Steele, H., Kennedy, R., Mattoon, G. et al. (1996). The relation of attachment status, psychiatric classification, and response to psychotherapy. *Journal of Consulting and Clinical Psychology, 64,* 22–31.

Fonagy, P., Roth, A., Steele, M., & Higgitt, A. (2005). The outcome of psychodynamic psychotherapy for psychological disorders. *Clinical Neuroscience Research Special Issue: Research in Psychoanalysis and Psychodynamics, 4,* 367–77.

Fonagy, P., Steele, H., & Steele, M. (1991). Maternal representations of attachment during pregnancy predict the organization of infant-mother attachment at one year of age. *Child Development, 62,* 891–905.

Fonagy, P., Steele, H., Moran, G., Steele, M., & Higgitt, A. (1991). The capacity for understanding mental states: The reflective self in parent and child and its significance for security of attachment. *Infant Mental Health Journal, 13,* 200–217.

Fraiberg, S. (1969). Libidinal object constancy and mental representation. *The Psychoanalytic Study of the Child, 24,* 9–47.

Fraiberg, S. (1980). *Clinical studies in infant mental health: The first year of life.* New York: Basic Books.

Freud, S. (1937). Analysis terminable and interminable. In J. Strachey (ed.), *The Standard Edition of the Complete Psychological Works of Sigmund Freud,* vol. 23, pp. 209–53. London: Hogarth Press.

Freud, A. (1965). *Normality and Pathology in Childhood: Assessments of Development.* Madison, CT: International Universities Press.

Friedman, L. (1988). The clinical polarity of object relations concepts. *Psychoanalytic Quarterly, LVII,* 667–91.

Frith, C. D. and Frith, U. (2006). The neural basis of mentalizing. *Neuron, 50*(4), 531–4.

Gabbard, G. and Westen, D. (2003). Rethinking therapeutic action. *International Journal of Psychoanalysis, 84*(4), 823–41.

Gabbard, G. O., Gunderson, J. G., & Fonagy, P. (2002). The place of psychoanalytic treatments within psychiatry. *Archives of General Psychiatry, 59,* 505–510.

Gellman, T., McKay, A. and Marks, L. (2010). Dynamic interpersonal therapy: providing a focus for time-limited psychodynamic work in the National Health Service. *Psychodynamic Therapy, 24,* 347–61.

Gerber, A. J., Kocsis, J. H., Milord, B. L., Roose, S. P., Barber, J. P., Thase, M. E., et al. (2011). A quality-based review of randomized controlled trials of psychodynamic psychotherapy. *Am J Psychiatry, 168*(1), 19–28.

Gill, M., & Hoffman, I. (1982). A method for studying the analysis of aspects of the patient's experience of the relationship in psychoanalysis and psychotherapy. *Journal of the American Psychoanalytic Association, 30,* 137–167.

Glass, R. M. (2008). Psychodynamic psychotherapy and research evidence: Bambi survives Godzilla? *Journal of the American Medical Association, 300*(13), 1587–9.

Glover, T. (1955). *Technique of Psychoanalysis.* New York: International University Press.

Goldberg, D. (2009). The interplay between biological and psychological factors in dete Psychoanal. *Psychother.,* 23, 236–47.

Greenberg, J. R., & Mitchell, S. A. (1983). *Object Relations in Psychoanalytic Theory.* Cambridge, MA: Harvard University Press.

Greenson, R. (1967). *The Technique and Practice of Psychoanalysis.* London: The Hogarth Press.

Gregory, R. J., Virk, S., Chlebowski, S., Kang, D., Remen, A. L., Soderberg, M. G. et al. (2008). A controlled trial of psychodynamic psychotherapy for co-occurring borderline personality disorder and alcohol use disorder. *Psychotherapy: Theory, Research, Practice, Training, 45*(1), 28–41.

Grunebaum, M. F., Galfalvy, H. C., Mortenson, L. Y., Burke, A. K., Oquendo, M. A., & Mann, J. J. (2010). Attachment and social adjustment: relationships to suicide attempt and major depressive episode in a prospective study. *J Affect Disord. 123*(1–3), 123–30.

Gunderson, A. and Gabbard, G. (1999). Making the case for psychoanalytic therapies. *Journal of the American Psychoanalytic Association, 47*, 679–704.

Hamill, M., Reid, M. and Reynolds, S. (2008). Letters in cognitive analytic therapy: the patient's experience. *Psychotherapy Research, 18*(5), 573–83.

Hammen, C. (2005). Stress and depression. *Annual Review of Clinical Psychology, 1*(1), 293–319.

Hazan, C. and Shaver, P. (1987). Romantic love conceptualized as an attachment process. *Journal of Personality and Social Psychology, 52*, 511–24.

Heim, C., Newport, D. J., Mletzko, T., Miller, A. H. and Nemeroff, C. B. (2008). The link between childhood trauma and depression: insights from HPA axis studies in humans. *Psychoneuroendocrinology, 33*(6), 693–710.

Hesse, P., & Cicchetti, D. (1982). Perspectives on an integrated theory of emotional development. *New Directions for Child Development, 16*, 3–48.

Hirschberg, L. (1993) Clinical interview with infants and their families. In C. Zeanah (ed.), *Handbook of Infant Mental Health*, pp. 173–91. New York: Guilford Press.

Howard, K. I., Kopta, S. M., Krause, M. S. and Orlinsky, D. E. (1986). The dose–effect relationship in psychotherapy. Special Issue: psychotherapy research. *American Psychologist, 41*, 159–64.

Huber, D., Denscherz, C., Gastner, J., Henrich, G. and Klug, G. (submitted). Psychodynamic long-term psychotherapies and cognitive-behavior therapy in comparison.

Ingrassia, A. (2003). The use of letters in NHS psychotherapy: a tool to help with engagement, missed sessions and endings. *British Journal of Psychotherapy, 19*, 355–66.

Inoue, Y., Tonooka, Y., Yamada, K. and Kanba, S. (2004). Deficiency of theory of mind in patients with remitted mood disorder. *Journal of Affective Disorders, 82*(3), 403–9.

Inoue, Y., Yamada, K. and Kanba, S. (2006). Deficit in theory of mind is a risk for relapse of major depression. *Journal of Affective Disorders, 95*(1–3), 125–7.

Insel, T. R. (2003). Is social attachment an addictive disorder? *Physiology and Behavior, 79*(3), 351–7.

Insel, T. R. and Wang, P. S. (2010). Rethinking mental illness. *Journal of the American Medical Association, 303*(19), 1970–1.

Insel, T., Cuthbert, B., Garvey, M., Heinssen, R., Pine, D. S. and Quinn, K. (2010). Research domain criteria (RDoC): toward a new classification framework for research on mental disorders. *American Journal of Psychiatry, 167*(7), 748–51.

Jefferys, D. B., Leakey, D., Lewis, J. A., Payne, S. and Rawlins, M. D. (1998). New active substances authorised in the United Kingdom between 1972 and 1994. *British Journal of Clinical Pharmacology, 45*, 151–6.

Jones, E. (1927). Discussion on lay analysis. *International Journal of Psychoanalysis, 8*, 174–98.

Joseph, B. (1983). On understanding and not understanding technical issues. *International Journal of Psychoanalysis, 64*, 139, 291–8.

Kaufman, J., Yang, B. Z., Douglas-Palumberi, H., Houshyar, S., Lipschitz, D., Krystal, J. H. et al. (2004). Social supports and serotonin transporter gene moderate depression in maltreated children. *Proceedings of the National Academy of Sciences USA, 101*(49), 17316–21.

Kazdin, A. E. (2006). Arbitrary metrics: implications for identifying evidence-based treatments. *American Psychologist, 61*(1), 42–9.

Kazdin, A. E. (2009). Understanding how and why psychotherapy leads to change. *Psychotherapy Research, 19*(4–5), 418–28.

Kernberg, O. F. (1975). *Borderline Conditions and Pathological Narcissism*. New York: Jason Aronson.

Kernberg, O. F. (1976a). Technical considerations in the treatment of borderline personality organization. *Journal of the American Psychoanalytic Association, 24*, 795–829.

Kernberg, O. F. (1976b). Foreword. In V. D. Volkan (Ed.), Primitive Internalized Object Relations (pp. xiii–xvii). New York: International Universities Press.

Kernberg, O. F. (1976c). *Object Relations Theory and Clinical Psychoanalysis*. New York: Aronson.

Kernberg, O. F. (1980). Internal World and External Reality: Object Relations Theory Applied. New York: Aronson.

Kernberg, O. F. (1982). Self, ego, affects and drives. *Journal of the American Psychoanalytic Association, 30*, 893–917.

Kernberg, O. F. (1985). *Internal World and External Reality: Object Relations Theory Applied*. New York: Aronson.

Kernberg, O. F. (1987). An ego psychology-object relations theory approach to the transference. *Psychoanalytic Quarterly, 51*, 197–221.

Kernberg, O. F., Clarkin, J. F. and Yeomans, F. E. (2006). *Transference Focused Psychotherapy for the Borderline Patient*. New York: Jason Aronson.

Kerr, N., Dunbar, R. I. M. and Bentall, R. P. (2003). Theory of mind deficits in bipolar affective disorder. *Journal of Affective Disorders, 73*(3), 253–9.

Kessler, R. C., Nelson, C. B., McGonagle, K. A., Liu, J., Swartz, M., & Blazer, D. G. (1996). Comorbidity of DSM-III-R major depressive disorder in the general population. *Br J Psychiatry, 168*, 17–30.

Kiesler, D. J. (1983). The 1982 interpersonal circle: a taxonomy for complementarity in human transactions. *Psychological Review, 90*, 185–214.

Kiesler, D. J. (1996). *Contemporary Interpersonal Theory and Research: Personality, Psychopathology, and Psychotherapy*. New York: Wiley.

Kirsner, D. (1990). Mystics and professionals in the culture of American psychoanalysis. *Free Associations, 20*, 85–104.

Klauber, J. (1981). *Difficulties in the Analytic Encounter*. London: Jason Aronson.

Klein, D. N., Schwartz, J. E., Santiago, N. J., Vivian, D., Vocisano, C., Castonguay, L. G. et al. (2003). Therapeutic alliance in depression treatment: controlling for prior change and patient characteristics. *Journal of Consulting and Clinical Psychology, 71*(6), 997–1006.

Klug, G. and Huber, D. (2009). Psychic structure: exploring an empirically still unknown territory. *Journal of the American Psychoanalytic Association, 57*(1), 149–73.

Knekt, P., Lindfors, O., Harkanen, T., Valikoski, M., Virtala, E., Laaksonen, M. A. et al. (2008). Randomized trial on the effectiveness of long- and short-term psychodynamic psychotherapy and solution-focused therapy on psychiatric symptoms during a 3-year follow-up. *Psychological Medicine, 38*(5), 689–703.

Knijnik, B., Blanco, C., Salum, M., Moraes C., Mombach, C, Almeida, E. et al. (2008). Pilot study of clonazepam versus psychodynamic group treatment plus clonazepam in the treatment of generalized social anxiety disorder. *European Psychiatry, 23*(8), 567–74.

Kopta, S. M., Lueger, R. J., Saunders, S. M. and Howard, K. I. (1999). Individual psychotherapy outcome and process research: challenges leading to greater turmoil or a positive transition? *Annual Review of Psychology, 50*, 441–69.

Korner, A., Gerull, F., Meares, R. and Stevenson, J. (2006). Borderline personality disorder treated with the conversational model: a replication study. *Comprehensive Psychiatry, 47*, 406–11.

Kramer, S., & Akhtar, S. (1988). The Developmental Context of Internalized Preoedipal Object Relations–Clinical Applications of Mahler's Theory of Symbiosis and Separation-Individuation. *Psychoanal. Q., 57*, 547–76.

Kriston, L., Holzel, L. and Harter, M. (2009). Analyzing effectiveness of long-term psychodynamic psychotherapy. *Journal of the American Medical Association, 301*(9), 930–1; author reply 32–3.

Kupfer, D. J. (1991). Long-term treatment of depression. *Journal of Clinical Psychiatry, 52*(Suppl. 5), 28–34.

Kyte, Z. A. and Goodyer, I. (2008). Social cognition in depressed children and adolescents. In C. Sharp, P. Fonagy, and I. Goodyer (eds), *Social Cognition and Developmental Psychopathology*, pp. 201–37. Oxford: Oxford University Press.

La Greca, A. M., Silverman, W. K. and Lochman, J. E. (2009). Moving beyond efficacy and effectiveness in child and adolescent intervention research. *Journal of Consulting and Clinical Psychology, 77*(3), 373–82.

Laupacis, A., Sackett, D. L. and Roberts, R. S. (1988). An assessment of clinically useful measures of the consequences of treatment. *New England Journal of Medicine, 318*(26), 1728–33.

Lear, J. (1993). An interpretation of transference. *International Journal of Psychoanalysis, 72*, 739–55.

Lee, A. and Hankin, B. L. (2009). Insecure attachment, dysfunctional attitudes, and low self-esteem predicting prospective symptoms of depression and anxiety during adolescence. *Journal of Clinical Child and Adolescent Psychology, 38*(2), 219–31.

Lee, L., Harkness, K. L., Sabbagh, M. A. and Jacobson, J. A. (2005). Mental state decoding abilities in clinical depression. *Journal of Affective Disorders, 86*(2–3), 247–58.

Leichsenring, F. and Rabung, S. (2008). Effectiveness of long-term psychodynamic psychotherapy: a meta-analysis. *Journal of the American Medical Association, 300*(13), 1551–65.

Leichsenring, F., Hoyer, J., Beutel, M., Herpertz, S., Hiller, W., Irle, E. et al. (2009). The Social Phobia Psychotherapy Research Network (SOPHO-NET)—the first multi-center randomized controlled trial of psychotherapy for social phobia: rationale, methods and patient characteristics. *Psychotherapy and Psychosomatics, 78*, 35–41.

Leichsenring, F., Masuhr, O., Jaeger, U., Dally, A., & Streeck, U. (2010). The effectiveness of psychoanalytic-interactional psychotherapy in borderline personality disorder. *Bull Menninger Clin, 74*(3), 206–18.

Leichsenring, F., Rabung, S. and Leibing, E. (2004). The efficacy of short-term psychodynamic psychotherapy in specific psychiatric disorders: a meta-analysis. *Archives of General Psychiatry, 61*, 1208–16.

Lemma, A. (2003). *Introduction to the Practice of Psychoanalytic Psychotherapy.* Chichester: Wiley.

Lemma, A. (in press). Some reflections on the 'teaching attitude' and its application to teaching about the use of the transference: a British view. *British Journal of Psychotherapy.*

Lemma, A. and Johnston, J. (2010). Editorial. *Psychoanalytic Psychotherapy: Applications, Theory, and Research, 24*(3), 179–82.

Lemma, A. and Patrick, M. (2010). Introduction. In *Off the Couch Contemporary Psychoanalytic Interpretation*, pp. 1–14. London: Routledge.

Lemma, A., Roth, A. and Pilling, S. (2008). The competences required to deliver effective psychoanalytic/psychodynamic therapy. Available at www.ucl.ac.uk/CORE (accessed 28/12/2010).

Lemma, A., Target, M. and Fonagy, P. (2010). The development of a brief psychodynamic protocol for depression: dynamic interpersonal therapy. *Psychoanalytic Psychotherapy: Applications, Theory and Research, 24*(4), 329–46.

Lewinsohn, P. M., Mischel, W., Chaplin, W. and Barton, R. (1980). Social competence and depression: the role of illusory self-perception. *Journal of Abnormal Psychology, 89*, 203–12.

Lilienfeld, S. O. (2007). Psychological treatments that cause harm. *Perspectives on Psychological Science, 2*, 53–70.

Loewald, H. (1986). Transference-countertransference. *Journal of the American Psychoanalytic Association, 34*, 275–88.

Luborsky, L., Diguer, L., Seligman, D. A., Rosenthal, R., Krause, E. D., Johnson, S. et al. (1999). The researcher's own therapy allegiances: a 'wild card' in comparisons of treatment efficacy. *Clinical Psychology: Science and Practice, 6*, 95–106.

Lussier, A. (1988). The limitations of the object relations model. *Psychoanalytic Quarterly, 57*, 528–46.

Luyten, P. and Blatt, S. J. (2007). Looking back towards the future: is it time to change the DSM approach to psychiatric disorders? The case of depression. *Psychiatry, 70*(2), 85–99.

Luyten, P., Blatt, S. J., Van Houdenhove, B. and Corveleyn, J. (2006). Depression research and treatment: are we skating to where the puck is going to be? *Clinical Psychology Review, 26*(8), 985–99.

Luyten, P., Corveleyn, J. and Blatt, S. J. (2005). The convergence among psychodynamic and cognitive-behavioral theories of depression: a critical overview of empirical research. In J. Corveleyn, P. Luyten and S. J. Blatt (eds), *The Theory and Treatment of Depression: Towards a Dynamic Interactionism Model*, pp. 107–47. Mahwah, NJ: Lawrence Erlbaum Associates.

Luyten, P., Fonagy, P., Lemma, A. and Target, M. (2011). Mentalizing and depression. In A. W. Bateman and P. Fonagy (eds), *Mentalizing in Mental Health Practice*, pp. xx. Washington, DC: American Psychiatric Press, Inc.

Luyten, P., Mayes, L., Fonagy, P. and Van Houdenhove, B. (2009). *The interpersonal regulation of stress.* Unpublished manuscript, University of Lueven.

Lynch, D., Laws. K. R., & McKenna, P. J. (2009). Cognitive behavioural therapy for major psychiatric disorder: Does it really work? A meta-analytical review of well controlled trials. *Psychological Medicine, 40*, 9–24.

McLaughlin, J. T. (1981). Transference, psychic reality and countertransference. *Psychoanalytic Quarterly, 50*, 639–664.

Main, M. (1991). Metacognitive knowledge, metacognitive monitoring, and singular (coherent) vs. multiple (incoherent) model of attachment: Findings and directions for future research. In C. M. Parkes, J. Stevenson-Hinde & P. Marris (Eds.), *Attachment Across the Life Cycle* (pp. 127–159). London: Tavistock/Routledge.

Main, M. and Goldwyn, R. (1998). *Adult attachment scoring and classification system.* Unpublished manuscript, University of California, Berkeley.

Main, M., Kaplan, N., & Cassidy, J. (1985). Security in infancy, childhood, and adulthood: A move to the level of representation. *Monographs of the Society for Research in Child Development, 50*(1–2), 66–104.

Maina, G., Forner, F. and Bogetto, F. (2005). Randomized controlled trial comparing brief dynamic and supportive therapy with waiting list condition in minor depressive disorders. *Psychotherapy and Psychosomatics, 74*, 3–50.

Malan, D., & Coughlin Della Selva, P. (2009). *Lives Transformed: An extremely powerful method of Short-term Dynamic Psychotherapy and its practical and theoretical significance.* London: Karnac Books.

Malhi, G., Adams, P., Porter, R., Wignall, A, Lampe, L., O'Connor, N., et al. (2009). Clinical practice recommendations for depression. *Acta Psychiatrica Scandinavica, 119*(Suppl. 439), 8–26.

Marziali, E. and Monroe-Blum, H. (1995). An interpersonal approach to group psychotherapy with borderline personality disorder. *Journal of Personality Disorders, 9*, 179–89.

Mason, A. (2000). Bion and binocular vision. *International Journal of Psychoanalysis, 81*, 983–9.

Masten, A. S. (1982). *Humor and Creative Thinking in Stress-Resistant Children,* University of Minnesota.

Michels, R. (1985). Perspectives on the nature of psychic reality: Panel introduction. *Journal of the American Psychoanalytic Association, 33*, 515–525.

Milrod, B., Busch, F., Cooper, A. and Shapiro, T. (1997). *Manual of Panic-focused Psychodynamic Psychotherapy.* Washington, DC: American Psychiatric Association Press.

Milrod, B., Leon, A. C., Busch, F., Rudden, M., Schwalberg, M., Clarkin, J. et al. (2007). A randomized controlled clinical trial of psychoanalytic psychotherapy for panic disorder. *American Journal of Psychiatry, 164*(2), 265–72.

Mitchell, S. A., & Black, M. (1995). *Freud and beyond.* New York: Basic Books.

Modell, A. (1990). *Other times, other realities.* Cambridge, MA: Harvard University Press.

Moffitt, T. E., Caspi, A., Harrington, H., Milne, B. J., Melchior, M., Goldberg, D. et al. (2007). Generalized anxiety disorder and depression: childhood risk factors in a birth cohort followed to age 32. *Psychological Medicine, 37*(3), 441–52.

Montag, C., Ehrlich, A., Neuhaus, K., Dziobek, I., Heekeren, H. R., Heinz, A. et al. (2010). Theory of mind impairments in euthymic bipolar patients. *Journal of Affective Disorders, 123*, 264–9.

Müller, C., Kaufhold, J., Overbeck, G. and Grabhorn, R. (2006). The importance of reflective functioning to the diagnosis of psychic structure. *Psychology and Psychotherapy, 79*(4), 485–94.

Neborsky, R. J. (2006). Brain, Mind and Dyadic Change Processes. *Journal of Clinical Psychology, 62*, 523–38.

Norcross, J. C., Hedges, M., & Castle, P. H. (2002). Psychologists conducting psychotherapy in 2001: A study of the Division 29 membership. *Psychotherapy, 39*, 97–102.

Ogden, T. H. (1992). Comments on transference and countertransference in the initial analytic meeting. *Psychoanalytic Inquiry, 12*, 225–47.

Okiishi, J. C., Lambert, M. J., Nielsen, S. L. and Ogles, B. M. (2003). Waiting for supershrink: an empirical analysis of therapist effects. *Clinical Psychology and Psychotherapy, 10*, 361–73.

Henri Poincar. "Hypotheses in Physics". Chapter 9 in *Science and Hypothesis,* London: Walter Scott Publishing (1905): p. 150.

Pressman, S. D. and Cohen, S. (2005). Does positive affect influence health? *Psychological Bulletin, 131*(6), 925–71.

Puschner, B., Kraft, S., Kachele, H. and Kordy, H. (2007). Course of improvement over 2 years in psychoanalytic and psychodynamic outpatient psychotherapy. *Psychology and Psychotherapy: Theory, Research and Practice, 80*(1), 51–68.

Rangell, L. (1985). On the theory of theory in psychoanalysis and the relation of theory to psychoanalytic therapy. *Journal of the American Psychoanalytic Association, 33*, 59–92.

Rawlins, M. (2008). *De Testimonio: On the Evidence for Decisions about the Use of Therapeutic Interventions.* London: Royal College of Physicians (The Harveian Oration).

Rinsley, D. B. (1977). An object relations view of borderline personality. In P. Hartocollis (Ed.), *Borderline personality disorders: The concept, the syndrome, the patient* (pp. 47–70). New York: International Universities Press.

Risch, N., Herrell, R., Lehner, T., Liang, K. Y., Eaves, L., Hoh, J. et al. (2009). Interaction between the serotonin transporter gene (*5-HTTLPR*), stressful life events, and risk of depression: a meta-analysis. *Journal of the American Medical Association, 301*(23), 2462–71.

Roback, H. B. (2000). Adverse outcomes in group psychotherapy: risk factors, prevention, and research directions. *Journal of Psychotherapy Practice and Research, 9*(3), 113–22.

Roepke, S. and Renneberg, B. (2009). Analyzing effectiveness of long-term psychodynamic psychotherapy. *Journal of the American Medical Association, 301*(9), 931–2; author reply 32–3.

Roth, A. and Fonagy, P. (2005). *What Works for Whom? A Critical Review of Psychotherapy Research*, 2nd edn. New York: Guilford Press.

Roth, A. D. and Pilling, S. (2008). Using an evidence-based methodology to identify the competences required to deliver effective cognitive and behavioural therapy for depression and anxiety disorders. *Behavioural and Cognitive Psychotherapy, 36*, 129–47.

Rustin, M. (2010). The complexities of service supervision: an experimental discovery. *Journal of child Psychotherapy, 36*, 3–15.

Ryle, A. (1990). *Cognitive Analytic Therapy: Active Participation in Change: New Integrations in Brief Psychotherapy.* Chichester: John Wiley and Sons.

Ryle, A. (2004). Writing by patients and therapists in cognitive analytic therapy. In G. Bolton, S. Howlett, C. Lago and J. Wright (eds), *Writing Cures: An Introductory Handbook of Writing, Counselling and Therapy*, pp. 59–71 London: Brunner-Routledge.

Sackett, D. L., Richardson, W. S., Rosenberg, W. M. and Haynes, R. B. (2000). *Evidence-based Medicine: How to Practice and Teach EBM*, 2nd edn. New York and Edinburgh: Churchill Livingstone.

Sackett, D. L., Rosenberg, W. M., Gray, J. A. M., Haynes, R. B. and Richardson, W. S. (1996). Evidence-based medicine: what it is and what it isn't. *British Medical Journal, 312*, 71–2.

Salminen, J. K., Karlsson, H., Hietala, J., Kajander, J., Aalto, S., Markkula, J., et al. (2008). Short-term psychodynamic psychotherapy and fluoxetine in major depressive disorder: A randomised comparative study. *Psychother Psychosom*, *77*, 351–57.

Sandler, J. (1987). *From safety to the superego: Selected papers of Joseph Sandler.* New York: Guilford Press.

Schafer, R. (1983). *The Analytic Attitude.* New York: Basic Books.

Schwaber, E. (1983). Psychoanalytic listening and psychic reality. *International Review of Psycho-Analysis*, *10*, 379–92.

Secretary of State for Health. (2008). *The Statement of Intent Made by the Minister for Health.* Paper presented at the Savoy Partnership Conference. Retrieved from http://www.iapt.nhs.uk/2008/12/statement-of-intent-november-2008/

Segal, H. (1993). Countertransference. In A. Alexandris and G. Vaslamatzis, (eds) *Countertransference: Theory, Technique, Teaching*, pp. 13–20. London: Karnac Books.

Shedler, J., Beck, A., Fonagy, P., Gabbard, G. O., Gunderson, J., Kernberg, O., et al. (2010). Personality Disorders in DSM-5. *American Journal of Psychiatry*, *167*(9), 1026–8.

Shedler, J., & Westen, D. (2004). Refining personality disorder diagnosis: integrating science and practice. *Am J Psychiatry*, *161*(8), 1350–1365.

Silove, D., Parker, G., Hadzi-Pavlovic, D., Maincavasagar, V., & Blaszczynski, A. (1991). Parental representations of patients with panic disorder and generalized anxiety disorder. *Br J Psychiatry*, *159*, 835–41.

Slade, A. (2000). The development and organisation of attachment: implications for pyschoanalysis. *Journal of the American Psychoanalytic Association, 48*(4), 1147–74.

Spruiell, V. (1988). The Indivisibility of Freudian Object Relations and Drive Theories. *Psychoanal. Q., 57*, 597–625.

Sroufe, L. A. (1996). *Emotional development: The organization of emotional life in the early years.* New York: Cambridge University Press.

Steiner, J. (2000). Containment, enactment and communication. *International Journal of Psychoanalysis, 81*, 245–55.

Stern, D. N. (1985). *The Interpersonal World of the Infant: A View from Psychoanalysis and Developmental Psychology.* New York: Basic Books.

Stolorow, R., Brandschaft, B., & Atwood, G. (1987). *Psychoanalytic treatment: An intersubjective approach.* Hillsdale, NJ: Analytic Press.

Strathearn, L., Fonagy, P., Amico, J. and Montague, R. (2009). Adult attachment predicts maternal brain and oxytocin response to infant cues. *Neuropsychopharmacology, 34*(13), 2655–66.

Strauss, S. E., Richardson, W. S., Glasziou, P. and Haynes, R. B. (2005). *Evidence-based Medicine: How to Practice and Teach EBM*, 3rd edn. New York: Elsevier.

Strenger, C. (1989). The classic and romantic visions in psychoanalysis. *International Journal of Psycho-Analysis, 70*, 595–610.

Sullivan, H. S. (1953). *The Interpersonal Theory of Psychiatry*. New York: Neston.

Srouge, L. A. (1996). *Emotional development the organization of emotional life in the early years*. New York: Cambridge University Press.

Svartberg, M., Stiles, T. C. and Seltzer, M. H. (2004). Randomized, controlled trial of the effectiveness of short-term dynamic psychotherapy and cognitive therapy for cluster C personality disorders. *American Journal of Psychiatry, 161*, 810–17.

Taylor, D. (2010). Psychoanalytic approaches and outcome research: Negative capability . . . Psychoanal. *Psychother., 24*, 398–416.

Terr, L. C. (1983). Chowchilla revisited: The effects of psychic trauma four years after a school-bus kidnapping. *American Journal of Psychiatry, 140*, 1543–1550.

Thombs, B. D., Bassel, M. and Jewett, L. R. (2009). Analyzing effectiveness of long-term psychodynamic psychotherapy. *Journal of the American Medical Association, 301*(9), 930; author reply 932–3.

Tolin, D. (2010). Is cognitive-behavioural therapy more effective than other therapies? A meta-analytic review. *Clin Psych Rev, 30*, 710–720.

Torgersen, S. (1986). Childhood and family characteristics in panic and generalised anxiety disorder. *American Journal of Psychiatry, 143*, 630–2.

Truant, G. S. (1999). Assessment of suitability for psychotherapy. II. Assessment based on basic process goals. *Am J Psychother, 53*(1), 17–34.

Tyrer, P., Tom, B., Byford, S., Schmidt, U., Jones, V., Davidson, K. et al. (2004). Differential effects of manual assisted cognitive behavior therapy in the treatment of recurrent deliberate self-harm and personality disturbance: the POPMACT study. *Journal of Personality Disorders, 18*(1), 102–16.

Ustun, T., Ayuso-Mateos, J., Chatterji, S., Mathers, C. and Murray, C. (2004). Global burden of depressive disorders in the year 2000+. *British Journal of Psychiatry, 184*, 386–92.

Van, H. L., Dekker, J., Koelen, J., Kool, S., van AAlst, G., Hendriksen, M., et al. (2009). Patient preference compared with random allocation in short-term psychodynamic supportive psychotherapy with indicated addition of pharmacotherapy for depression. *Psychotherapy Research, 19*(2), 205–212.

Van Houdenhove, B. and Luyten, P. (2009). Central sensitivity syndromes: stress system failure may explain the whole picture. *Seminars in Arthritis and Rheumatism, 39*(3), 218–19; author reply 220–1.

van IJzendoorn, M. H. (1995). Adult attachment representations, parental responsiveness, and infant attachment: a meta-analysis on the predictive validity of the Adult Attachment Interview. *Psychological Bulletin, 117*, 387–403; author reply 220–1.

Van Overwalle, F. (2009). Social cognition and the brain: a meta-analysis. *Human Brain Mapping, 30*(3), 829–58.

Wampold, B. E. (2001). *The Great Psychotherapy Debate: Models, Methods, and Findings*. Hillsdale, NJ: Laurence Erlbaum Associates.

Wampold, B. E., Imel, Z. E. and Minami, T. (2007). The story of placebo effects in medicine: evidence in context. *Journal of Clinical Psychology, 63*(4), 379–90.

Weiss, A. P., Guidi, J. and Fava, M. (2009). Closing the efficacy–effectiveness gap: translating both the what and the how from randomized controlled trials to clinical practice. *Journal of Clinical Psychiatry, 70*(4), 446–9.

Weissman, M., Markowitz, J. and Klerman, G (2000). *Comprehensive Guide to Interpersonal Psychotherapy*. New York: Basic Books.

Westen, D. (1989). Are 'primitive' object relations really preoedipal? *American Journal of Orthopsychiatry, 69*, 331–45.

Westen, D. and Bradley, R. (2005). Empirically supported complexity: rethinking evidence-based practice in psychotherapy. *Current Directions in Psychological Science, 14*(5), 266–71.

Westen, D., Novotny, C. M. and Thompson-Brenner, H. (2004). The empirical status of empirically supported psychotherapies: assumptions, findings, and reporting in controlled clinical trials. *Psychological Bulletin, 130*, 631–63.

Whalley, H. C., McKirdy, J., Romaniuk, L., Sussman J., Johnstone, E. C., Wan, H., and Hali, J. (2009). Functional imaging of emotional memory in bipolar disorder and schizophrenia. *Bipolar Disorders, 11*(80), 840–56.

Winnicott, D. W. (1962). Ego integration in child development. In D. W. Winnicott (ed.), *The maturational processes and the facilitating environment* (pp. 56–63). London: Hogarth Press, 1965.

Winnicott, D. W. (1965). *Maturational Processes and the Facilitating Environment*. London: Hogarth Press.

Winnicott, D. W. (1971). *Playing and Reality*. London: Tavistock Publications.

Yonkers, K. A., Warshaw, M. G., Massion, A. O., & Keller, M. B. (1996). Phenomenology and course of generalized anxiety disorder. *Br J Psychiatry, 168*(3), 308–13.

Index

Page numbers in *italic* indicate boxes, figures, and tables.

Printed and bound by CPI Group (UK) Ltd, Croydon, CR0 4YY